ALZHEIMER'S
A CAREGIVER'S GUIDE AND SOURCEBOOK

Howard Gruetzner, M.Ed.

Director, Regional Aging Services
Heart of Texas Region MHMR Center

WILEY

John Wiley & Sons, Inc.
New York • Chichester • Brisbane • Toronto • Singapore

Publisher: Stephen Kippur
Editor: David Sobel
Managing Editor: Ruth Greif
Editing, Design, and Production: Publications Development Co.

This publication is provided to serve the reader as a supplement to professional medical guidance and treatment, and not as a substitute for professional medical care. As new medical research broadens our knowledge, changes in treatment and drug therapy are required. The author and publisher have made every effort to ensure that information regarding medical treatment is accurate and in accordance with the standards accepted at the time of publication. Readers are advised, however, to follow the product information sheet included with any drug administered and to seek professional advice before proceeding with medical treatment.

This book was sponsored by

Heart of Texas Region Mental Health Mental Retardation, Waco, Texas
and
DePaul Center (A division of Providence Hospital, Daughters of Charity of St. Vincent DePaul), Waco, Texas

Library of Congress Cataloging-in-Publication Data

Gruetzner, Howard.
    Alzheimer's : a caregiver's guide and sourcebook.

    Bibliography: p. 231
    1. Alzheimer's disease.   I. Title.
RC523.G78 1988   362.1′9683   87-37249
ISBN 0-471-60082-2
ISBN 0-471-52203-1 (pbk.)

Printed in the United States of America

    10 9 8 7 6 5

To Bob Herbert,
a dedicated warrior for the welfare
of the community and its people.

CONTENTS

9   How to Respond Positively to Alzheimer's Behaviors   101

10 Exploring Community Resources   127

     Community Resources for Alzheimer's Care   131
     Considerations for Nursing Home Care   133
     Final Resource Considerations   138

PART II   RESEARCH AND TREATMENT   141

11 Abnormal Changes in the Brain   143

     Physical Changes in the Brain   144
     Anatomy of the Brain   145
     Neurofibrillary Tangles   148
     Senile or Neuritic Plaques   152
     Granulovacuolar Degeneration   156
     Hirano Bodies   158
     Congophilic Angiopathy   159
     Chemical Changes in the Brain   161
     More about Brain Anatomy   161
     The Cholinergic System   165
     The Serotonergic System   168
     The Noradrenergic System   169
     Somatostatin   169
     Treating Neurotransmitter Deficiencies   170
     Summary   171

12 Treatment Possibilities   172

     Should You Participate in Drug-Research
       Study?   174
     Inconsistencies in Drug Studies   175
     Cholinergic Agents   177
     Cholinergic Receptor Agonists   183
     Naxolone and Naltrexone   184
     Vasodilators and Nootropic Agents   185
     Neuropeptides   187

PREFACE

In the United States today, there are an estimated two million victims of Alzheimer's disease, and the number is growing. The disease eventually renders the brain virtually useless, and it turns lives inside out—both the lives of the people who have Alzheimer's and the lives of those closest to them. It is a slow, as yet irreversible, process that ultimately leads to death.

However, families confronted with Alzheimer's disease no longer must struggle through this difficult illness alone. Tremendous advances have been made in recent years in understanding the disease and devising successful care and management techniques—information that is presented in friendly layman's terms in *ALZHEIMER'S: A Caregiver's Guide and Sourcebook*. With this book as a companion, caring for an Alzheimer's patient can be a far more positive experience than families could have thought possible.

This book can give both families and professionals a better understanding of the disease, of the victim's behavior, and of ways to cope effectively with the demands of caring for Alzheimer's patients. The first ten chapters, based primarily on the author's ten years of specialized work with the elderly mentally-ill population in Central Texas, cover symptoms and stages of Alzheimer's and provide an overview of what to expect as the illness progresses. A special section explores the full range of resources for Alzheimer's care available in a community—resources that can provide families with much-appreciated relief from the burdens of daily care. The book also includes tips on locating resources such as diagnoses, home health services, and nursing home placements, as well as helpful suggestions on reducing caregiver stress.

Possible causes of Alzheimer's disease are considered in Part I. This discussion also addresses psychosocial factors that relate to this illness. Research is beginning to make some progress that broadens our knowledge of Alzheimer's. Other aspects of research are considered in Part II. Two of the book's last three chapters are designed to acquaint both caregivers and professionals with what actually happens in the brain as Alzheimer's disease progresses. Overviews of current drug treatment research, as well as other research findings which may contribute to treatment, are included for the reader.

Care management of the dementia patient can often benefit from careful use of traditional psychiatric medications. These medications, by providing helpful ways to reduce behavioral and emotional manifestations of the disease, may also extend the period of time the affected individual can be cared for in the home appropriately. With an understanding of care management principles outlined in this book and active utilization of existing resources, caregivers will be better equipped to cope with the physical and emotional challenge confronting them. Psychiatric medications are best used in this broader context of caregiving.

It is hoped that this guide will serve as a comprehensive reference that will make the caregiver's tasks easier, more rewarding, and more constructive. In turn, we hope it will help to make the lives of those caught in the grip of Alzheimer's disease happier, safer, and more comfortable.

ACKNOWLEDGMENTS

I am especially grateful to family, personal friends, and professional colleagues who gave their support to this book. Observing the challenges of caring for a relative with dementia has been both revealing and rewarding. Much more information than ever before is available now for families caring for loved ones who have Alzheimer's disease. When I began to work with people who had dementia in the early 1970s, the attitudes toward dementia were reflective of the negative social attitudes we had toward our aging citizens. It was not a comprehensive, sensitive approach to evaluation and treatment.

I am indebted to the staff of a local psychiatric hospital, De Paul Center, a division of Providence Hospital, Daughters of Charity of St. Vincent de Paul, and the psychiatrists associated with that hospital who provided helpful comments on the manuscript. The psychiatrists who took time to read the manuscript and comment include: Stephen Mark, M.D.; Bergen Morrison, M.D.; Thomas Stidvent, M.D.; and Jack Wentworth, M.D. I also appreciate other encouraging comments from Rod Ryan, M.D., Family Practice physician.

Dennis Myers, Ph.D., of the Baylor University Institute of Gerontological Studies used the section dealing with matters relevant to caregiving in a mental health and aging course. I appreciate Dr. Myers' comments and those of his students regarding the book's usefulness as a text. Martie Sauter of the McLennan Community College Mental Health Associates Degree Program was very generous in describing the book's usefulness for training students and caregivers.

To make the chapters dealing with scientific studies on research and treatment comprehensible and meaningful required considerable simplification. One risk of simplifying such material is that its accuracy may be compromised. I appreciate the comments made by a number of physicians including a neurosurgeon, R.H. Saxton, M.D.; a neurologist, Mark Schwartze, M.D.; a Family Practice physician, Edward Cooney, M.D.; a radiologist, R.L. Zeigler, M.D. The comments of Charles Conley, M.D., a pathologist, were extremely helpful in the sections involving plaques, tangles, and so forth. Bill Kersh, a biologist, reviewed sections concerning the chemical changes in the brain.

Hazel Limback, Deputy Executive Director of Heart of Texas Council of Governments, Area Agency on Aging gave consistent support and encouragement to this project. I appreciate her concern for persons affected by Alzheimer's disease and their needs. I also appreciate the interest shown by planners from the State of Texas, Office of the Governor and Texas Department of Aging concerning the special needs created by this disease.

Danny Fred provided tireless assistance with typing, rewriting, and editing. One of my colleagues, Samantha Anderson, provided helpful assistance with the editing and rewriting. Jeanne Levy spent extra hours typing the first draft of the section on research and treatment, which no doubt seemed to have been written in a foreign language. I appreciate other typing assistance from a friend, Pam Richard, R.N., who unselfishly provided her time and support.

Katherine Gregor edited the final manuscript with professional objectivity, clarity, and sensitivity. Lynn Pearson provided tireless assistance with typing, rewriting, and editing for the entire book. She was especially helpful in keeping the manuscript simple and readable.

Staff of MHMR Aging Services provided more support than they know in attending to the needs of our clients. I appreciate these ladies: Vanessa Hummel, Terry Brandon, Melissa Talamantes, and Melba Ogle.

I am pleased to have had the opportunity to work with clients, families, and the Waco-area Alzheimer's Family Support Group. These persons openly revealed their lives and encouraged the writing of this book, realizing that it could help others as well as themselves. This book is for caregivers whose commitment to their loved ones with Alzheimer's disease teaches us all something more about the meaning of personal sacrifice and human courage.

Three people were instrumental in guiding this manuscript toward publication. I want to express my special thanks to these persons and their respective organizations: Anthony V. Klucznik, Word Publishing, Waco, Texas; Nancy Marcus Land, Publications Development Co., Crockett, Texas. Finally, I wish to thank David Sobel of John Wiley & Sons, Inc., for his direction in improving what we had started.

SPECIAL ACKNOWLEDGMENT

About the Poetry

MAUDE NEWTON has survived one of the most difficult experiences life can hand a person: watching her husband, Frank, move slowly, progressively toward death. Frank Newton, who had retired from a successful career in banking, real estate, and insurance in Del Rio, TX. had Alzheimer's disease.

As Mrs. Newton went through all of the disease's stages with her husband, she began an intimate chronicle of her thoughts and feelings in verse form.

"I started picking up whatever was handy—the backs of envelopes, notepaper, whatever—to write about how I was feeling at that moment," she said. "I found it was doing me a lot of good. I was verbalizing my feelings, even if just on a piece of paper." Her children insisted she save all her scribbled thoughts; later, they typed, copied, and bound the collection. Mrs. Newton's poetry introduces a number of issues in a personal, moving way, and we thank her for allowing us to reprint a few of her poems.

Part I
THE CAREGIVER EXPERIENCE

Alzheimer's disease cannot be cured. Part I focuses on what we know about this disease and what we can do to care for individuals thought to have Alzheimer's. A better understanding of this condition and its behavioral manifestations enables caregivers to respond more effectively to the needs of loved ones.

Our beliefs about the Alzheimer's patient and his behavior do not take into account the effects of brain impairment. We have no frame of reference through which brain-impaired behavior can be understood. Part I provides this perspective so that caregivers can more effectively and positively respond to the problems and needs of their loved ones.

The caregiver experience is characterized by the adjustment of the Alzheimer's patient and his family to this illness. Part I will examine this adjustment in several ways. Stages of the illness and the family adjustment will be considered. A step-by-step guide describes the experience from the time initial symptoms are noticed to the point care is planned and caregiver stress encountered. Practical approaches to these steps are considered. Community resources are described in the last chapter of Part I since social support is such an important way for caregivers to provide for the increasing needs of their loved ones and themselves.

TWILIGHT

It's that time again,
that time when day fades into night . . .
that time when—
if you were working late
(and I had a few minutes to wait),
I'd pick up the papers on the floor,
fluff up the pillows a bit,
and open the door to look for you.
It was good to sit on the sofa
and feel you close—
to hear about your day
and share mine with you.

It was always my favorite time of the day
when the bustle gave way
to the shared things we used to say.

Now I dread it—
I hate to sit and watch it come on—
without you.
It's just a time I must learn to endure—
to live through.

Maude S. Newton

1

WHAT IS ALZHEIMER'S DISEASE?

A case history Jewell Johnson had once been quite active in her neighborhood. She had also attended church regularly. These activities had not significantly changed following her husband's death three years earlier. Her friends and family had been impressed with how well she made it through the grief and kept her life going. She had always been stronger and healthier than her husband. Mrs. Johnson was now 74 and seemed to be a model for aging.

Uncharacteristic behavior is noticed. Several months ago her closest neighbors began to notice changes. First, she dropped out of church. They discovered that her feelings had been hurt. Apparently, she had made some mistakes as the treasurer of her Sunday School class, losing several hundred dollars. That was not her story, though; Mrs. Johnson insisted that someone had stolen the money. It had all been cash, and for some reason she had never deposited it in the bank.

She began to stay home more and more often. It also surprised the neighbors that she discouraged their visits. They were becoming worried about her and considered calling relatives, but her son and daughter both lived several hundred miles away and telephoned regularly. Their professional jobs made it difficult to visit very often. The pastor tried to visit, but Jewell was uncharacteristically rude to him and other church members who tried to visit her.

3

Household chores and personal hygiene are neglected.

The yard was still covered with leaves left since the fall. It was now the middle of winter. On occasion, neighbors would check on Jewell. Several times a week her morning newspapers remained in the yard, and this gave neighbors an excuse to check on her. She always came to the door in her robe and slippers. She thanked them for the paper, making excuses that she had a cold and was resting more. She refused their offers to help her. If they pursued these offers too long, she would become more restless and agitated. A few times she had shut the door abruptly.

Her closest next-door neighbor called the daughter, Joan. Joan was caught off guard because the phone conversations with her mother—while briefer and more vague—had not been that different. Her mother had always been self-reliant and independent; it was no surprise that she was so reluctant to accept help. It was strange that Jewell never told her daughter of any problems. Maybe that was why the conversations were briefer and so general. The neighbor was asked to watch after Jewell, and the daughter called her mother.

Behavior changes are denied.

This was not a pleasant conversation, nor was it very long. Jewell denied any problems and told her daughter the neighbor was meddling. Jewell thought the neighbor's son was trying to get her house. The next-door neighbor had never been honest. As the paranoia became more vivid, Jewell became more upset and hung up on the daughter. Joan called the neighbor and said she would be down the following weekend.

Bills remain unpaid.

The next day both the gas and electric company cut off their services to Jewell's home. In the dead of winter, they do not usually cut off the services of elderly people. The neighbor argued on Jewell's behalf but to no avail. She had not paid her bills for more than three months (about the same time she stopped attending church). Attempts to get Mrs. Johnson to the door failed. She would look out the window briefly, but that was all she would do. No one could get into the house. Neighbors called the daughter, but they could think of nothing else that would help.

Delusions develop. Late that night, the neighbors were awakened by screaming outside Jewell's house. It was nearly freezing, and she was outside her home in a gown. She was afraid of the neighbors who tried to help calm her. She kept talking about her husband roaming around in the attic. She was afraid of him. The police were called and when they arrived on the scene, Mrs. Johnson was frightened and still very upset. She was quite confused and could only talk about her husband in the attic. They investigated and found no sign of anyone in the attic—just as they had expected. A crisis hot line was called, and Mrs. Johnson was hospitalized since she had become a danger to herself.

Closer examination of the household was revealing. There was not any food in the household. She probably had not eaten anything to speak of for several days. The kitchen was a mess, and the gas burners were still turned on although gas service had been terminated. The police explored the rest of the household. Clothes were lying around. The toilet had not been flushed for days, and Mrs. Johnson had had some accidents in her bedroom. Newspapers lay on the living room floor rolled up and unread. Bills and other mail were heaped in piles near the newspapers.

After being stabilized in the psychiatric hospital, a thorough examination was conducted. Upon its completion, only one conclusion could explain what had happened to Mrs. Jewell Johnson over the past year to six months. Something had obviously been happening before her behavior changes suggested something was wrong. In fact, it was admirable that she had so successfully compensated for the difficulties she was experiencing in memory and thinking. The diagnosis was inescapable—probable Alzheimer's disease.

It was 1980, and her family and friends were bewildered. They had never heard of Alzheimer's disease. They had been prepared to accept a diagnosis of "senility." Maybe her problems could be explained by depression or old age. The friends of Jewell Johnson and her family began to try to understand what was happening and what would be done.

Alzheimer's disease? That sounds so strange and terrible. What is Alzheimer's disease?

Alzheimer's disease is a condition of unknown origin that causes gradual loss of abilities in memory, thinking, reasoning, judgment, orientation, and concentration. Alzheimer's disease is not the result of normal aging, but it does occur more frequently in persons who are 65 years of age or older.

More than simple forgetfulness   Alzheimer's disease is far more serious than the occasional forgetfulness experienced by the elderly. In its early stages, however, the disease can be difficult to distinguish from ordinary forgetfulness. The disease affects the brain gradually, and persons ordinarily will compensate for the early symptoms; thus neither the victim nor those around her may suspect a medical problem at first. The results of Alzheimer's slow but progressive damage to the brain often are not noticed until the person experiences greater than normal stress, pressures, or losses that stretch her coping abilities to the breaking point, or until the damage to the brain reaches an advanced stage.

Causes of disease unknown   Although much is known about the symptoms of the disease, little is known of the causes. Ongoing research is being conducted toward unlocking the secret of the disease, but at present neither a full scientific understanding nor a cure exists.

Research has revealed differences in the brains of persons with this disease such as abnormal proteins and higher concentrations of aluminum. Nonetheless, it is not known whether these abnormalities are a cause or result of the disease process. Since there is no cure, treatment consists of symptom management and overall care of the person.

The disease was first identified in 1906 by a German neurologist, Alois Alzheimer (pronounced Altz-hi-merz). His subject was a 51-year-old woman who exhibited problems with memory and disorientation. Later, Alzheimer identified depression and hallucinations as additional symptoms. The woman's condition continued to deteriorate; a severe dementia was evident, and the woman eventually died. An autopsy of the woman revealed that her brain had cortical atrophy and abnormalities in the cerebral cortex called neurofibrillary tangles. These changes in the brain were thought to have caused the impairment of the woman's memory, her disorientation, and her cognitive and emotional decline.

Two million people in the United States affected

Initially, Alzheimer's disease was considered rare and was believed to occur only in people under age 60. We now know that the disease is not rare, and that it in fact occurs most frequently in the older population. Of the more than 22 million persons in the United States now over 65, an estimated 5 percent to 7 percent, or about two million persons, are thought to have Alzheimer's. The incidence increases further with age; Alzheimer's strikes about 20 percent of people over age 80.

Alzheimer's disease is the most common neurological disease that causes dementia, a brain condition that results in a loss of intellectual capacities and impairs both social and occupational functioning. The incidence of the disease in women is a little higher than in men. As the life span of males increases, these differences in incidence will decrease. The disease knows no socioeconomic boundaries. Once persons develop Alzheimer's, their life expectancy is reduced by approximately one-third. However, the severity of the dementia and the rate of deterioration vary with the individual. Other health factors naturally contribute to life expectancy in the presence of Alzheimer's. Death is often attributed to respiratory conditions that develop in the late stages of Alzheimer's.

As elderly population grows, more persons are affected.

The number of persons with Alzheimer's disease is expected to increase in the next decades as the elderly population increases. The disease is estimated to be the fourth or fifth leading cause of death in the United States, killing more than 100,000 persons annually. Studies have indicated that up to 58 percent of the nation's nursing home population is afflicted with Alzheimer's, although many of these persons have never been diagnosed as Alzheimer's victims.

WHY?

I've heard it said,
"If there weren't a God
we would invent one,
for in our hour of deepest need
we must have someone—
some power on which to call."

I don't know . . .
I try hard to believe—
but we are rational creatures.
I must think,
or why was I given a mind?

I think and think
and it makes no sense.
Why would a loving Father
do this to my mate?
Why would he take from him
his mind—his pride
in being alive?

Why would he rob from him
his joy in being here?
Why leave him thus—
a poor shambling caricature
of the man he was?

Surely not for my sake—
to test my power to believe.
If so, it has defeated its purpose.
It's left me tormented and vulnerable
seeking an answer—and finding none—
and calling out—
"Oh, God—if you are my God, Why?"

Maude S. Newton

2
SYMPTOMS AND PHASES OF ALZHEIMER'S DISEASE

Symptoms of Alzheimer's Disease

Alzheimer's disease: a neurological condition causing deficient thinking and remembering

Alzheimer's disease is a neurological condition that impairs the brain's functioning. (Its exact cause is not known, but the leading theories will be explored in Chapters 4 and 11.) Symptoms of the illness represent deficits in many areas of how a person remembers and thinks. For instance, problems with memory may be manifested as forgetting names, dates, places, whether a bill has been paid, or something said over and over. Intellectual abilities are lost eventually. Reasoning with the affected person is no longer a successful way to understand and deal with his problems. Judgment about common everyday situations is drastically diminished. The individual's capacity to express himself verbally gradually shrinks. Neither is he able to comprehend what others say to him. As the disease progresses, he may gradually lose the ability to speak. Psychiatric symptoms such as delusions and hallucinations can occur. The person can become anxious, restless, agitated, and may even appear to be depressed. His personality will change. In fact, he may not seem to be the same person. What kind of disease is Alzheimer's disease?

Alzheimer's disease produces symptoms that are characteristic of a syndrome known as *dementia.* This type of condition was inaccurately labeled in the past as senility by both professionals and the public when older persons became forgetful and were unable to adequately care for themselves. A more general term still in use for

9

dementia is "organic brain syndrome." Organic brain syndrome is a general diagnostic term, whereas senility is a catch-all, wastebasket kind of term that reflects attitudes about aging instead of a diagnostic impression.

Dementia: loss of intellectual abilities

Dementia, in its broader sense, indicates a loss or impairment of a person's abilities to use his mind. The essential feature of dementia is a loss of intellectual abilities severe enough to interfere with social or occupational functioning. An accountant with Alzheimer's disease will be unable to perform his job because of impairments in memory, reasoning, and calculation abilities. A farmer will become unable to plant and harvest crops. Buying seed and figuring out how much seed to put in planters or drills will become impossible.

Alzheimer's disease is the most common type of dementia that affects older persons. It is not, however, the only dementing illness that affects this population. Multiple strokes can create a dementia that resembles Alzheimer's disease. Depression and other psychiatric illnesses can also produce conditions similar to dementia. These psychiatric conditions, especially depression, are often referred to as pseudodementia or "false" dementia because, while they create similar symptoms, the underlying cause is different. Some conditions that cause symptoms of dementia can be healed. This is true, for example, of B-12 deficiencies, thyroid disturbances, and pernicious anemia. Usually proper treatment will reverse the symptoms of such false dementias.

Other causes of the dementia must first be ruled out.

At this time there is no definitive medical test that can diagnose Alzheimer's disease. Other potential causes of dementia must be ruled out. This is extremely important, not only to arrive at a correct diagnosis, but to identify any treatable condition. The coexistence of several conditions may cause dementia. Even if one condition, such as Alzheimer's disease, cannot be treated in the sense of cured or slowed, it is important to treat the conditions which can be managed. The treatment will very likely improve the individual's functioning to some degree, despite the fact that he has a progressive dementing illness.

Alzheimer's disease is a probable diagnosis given only after all other potential causes of dementia have been identified and treated or ruled out. Alzheimer's disease may also be referred to as a primary degenerative dementia. For professionals, more specific discussion of these clinical criteria can be found in the *Diagnostic and Statistical Manual of Mental Disorders* (see Bibliography). The onset of the Alzheimer's-type dementia can also be specified. Presenile onset means the disease process began by age 65 or before; senile onset indicates that the condition began after age 65.

We will now consider the symptoms that constitute a dementing illness like Alzheimer's disease, particularly the everyday manifestations of symptoms. Since special psychological tests are often used to identify or confirm some of these symptoms, the applications to everyday situations are not always clearly made. We will follow the basic diagnostic criteria established in DSM III. For more specifics, the reader may refer to the "Behavior Profile" in the appendix. It lists many symptomatic manifestations of diagnostic criteria for a dementia like Alzheimer's disease.

First criteria for dementia: severe loss of intellectual functioning

The first criteria for dementia is the *loss of intellectual abilities* of sufficient severity to interfere with social or occupational functioning. This indicates that not only are these abilities impaired, but they also must be affected to the degree that the person cannot perform usual work-related activities satisfactorily. For instance, a teacher will be unable to prepare lessons and keep his presentations to the class organized and comprehensible. He may be unable to provide information that was very easy for him to grasp before the Alzheimer's process began. New academic demands may become quite stressful. In social situations he may have trouble following conversations and become confused by new points of discussion. Social demands can become more troublesome, and he may withdraw or become more anxious in social situations. His responses to other people may make less sense and not be very well related to a topic of conversation.

Routine activities become increasingly difficult.

As Alzheimer's disease progresses, a person's ability to successfully carry out familiar activities of daily living will decline. The thinking abilities required to cook a meal, pay bills, clean house, bathe, dress, or even dial a telephone will diminish gradually. Because of memory problems, the person may also claim that tasks have been done, although it is quite evident they have not.

Severe memory problems are often the earliest symptoms.

Memory impairment has many manifestations during the course of Alzheimer's disease. Forgetfulness is often listed as a condition of old age, and in fact some memory loss is normal in later years. Misplacing keys or a checkbook is something all of us have experienced, regardless of our age. The memory impairment that occurs with Alzheimer's disease is much more pervasive and disabling. Problems with memory are usually the earliest and most obvious symptom of this condition. It is also a symptom that is often denied by individuals with Alzheimer's disease.

Ability to remember recently received information is affected first.

Recent memory, that is, memory for events and information experienced over the past half hour, is most affected earlier in Alzheimer's. Such memory loss obviously affects a person's daily living circumstances. Bills are not paid, the gas may be left on, appointments are missed, or keeping track of a daily routine is disturbed. Immediate recall is the ability to repeat something that has just been said. Persons with Alzheimer's disease may have good immediate recall, but little information is likely to be remembered later. New information is not easily remembered.

New learning affected

Recent memory problems also make it difficult for persons with an Alzheimer's-type dementia to learn new material or activities. For example, keeping up with time and place, learning new names, or remembering a shopping list, which involve recent memory abilities, become increasingly difficult as the disease progresses. Disorientation, which involves forgetting time, person, and place, can occur in Alzheimer's disease. For example, the person will reach a point when he cannot remember the day of the week, the month, or the year. Such disorientation and memory problems will contribute to the person's getting lost and will be especially evident in new situations or places.

Memories of past remain longer. Remote memory is the person's grasp of his past. For instance, this involves information about where he was born, when he was born, his parents and siblings, where he attended school, and when he graduated from school. Personal history is recorded in remote memory. Remote memory also includes facts about past presidents, wars, economic, and political events. In the early stages of Alzheimer's disease, remote memory is less obviously affected but becomes more noticeably impaired over time. Direct questions or confrontations will expose gaps that exist in remote memory. Distant memories may serve as a refuge when recent memory becomes so severely affected the individual cannot relate to what is currently happening.

Maintenance of daily routines is helpful for memory-impaired persons. Such routines can help organize a life that has become unpredictable and insecure because failing memory cannot assist the individual in controlling daily events and interactions.

The loss of intellectual functioning and impaired memory are essential ingredients in an Alzheimer's-type dementia, but several other symptoms of dementia must also be present. Some of these do not occur until later in the course of the illness and may vary considerably from one person to the next. At least one of the following symptoms must be present for primary degenerative dementia to be diagnosed.

Faulty judgment puts Alzheimer's patients in dangerous situations *Impaired judgment and insight* are symptoms which are manifested in the lives of persons with Alzheimer's disease. Impaired judgment occurs in many areas of the person's life and can lead to dangerous consequences. For example, the person may insist on driving the car when it is clear his ability has been seriously impaired. He may insist he can manage his finances as well as anyone, even when obviously he cannot. Cooking and lighting stoves are activities where poor judgment may become evident as well as dangerous.

Of course, the dementing process is responsible for impaired judgment. However, some environments encourage rather than restrict the exercise of poor judgment. Some caregivers may be understandably anxious about confronting these kinds of behaviors, but the need to intervene usually increases with the potential risks to the Alzheimer's patient, especially when they carry with them risks to other persons. (Driving is a good example of this type of situation.)

Abilities to discern differences and similarities between things decrease.

Impairment of abstract thinking is more difficult to recognize in everyday actions. It is more easily assessed by answers to certain types of questions. For example, proverbs such as "Haste makes waste" are difficult for persons with dementia to adequately explain. The similarities and differences between things cannot be discerned. A chair and desk are alike because both are furniture. Such associations are not likely to be made by the person with Alzheimer's disease. Defining words and concepts are other examples of tasks that require abstract thinking or reasoning.

Alzheimer's disease affects the cortex of the brain. The cortex is discussed more specifically in Chapter 11, but we should make one point here. There are several human functions controlled by the cortex, the brain's outer layer. Some of these functions involve speech and movement abilities.

Aphasia, a problem with speaking and understanding language, develops.

One disturbance of cortical functioning associated with Alzheimer's disease is called *aphasia.* Aphasia is the loss of previously possessed abilities in language comprehension or production. Because of damage to the brain, an individual is unable to understand speech. Verbal expression also becomes disturbed in Alzheimer's disease.

These speech deficits do not occur abruptly, as is common with a stroke. Speech abilities are gradually eroded. Individual variations occur during the disease process, but usually speech problems begin with some difficulty in word-finding. When talking, the person may have trouble making a point or answering a question directly. Spontaneous speech can be wordy and evasive. His comments wander around the point but never get to it. Later, word-finding problems and inability to name objects become very apparent.

Comprehension of what others say becomes impaired; thus the person is reluctant to engage in conversation. Spoken words or combinations of words are also misused. Later, even misused words have less meaningful relationships to the words for which they are substituted. The person may even echo what is said to him. Finally, the ability to produce sounds and words is reduced because the person is having difficulty coordinating his speech apparatus. The complete inability to speak will occur in many persons during the very last stage of Alzheimer's disease.

Difficulties in performing purposeful movement, apraxia, become evident.

Additionally, difficulties in movement can occur with Alzheimer's disease. One such impairment of movement is called *apraxia*. Apraxia is the loss of a previously possessed ability to perform skilled and purposeful motor acts. It is not the result of weakness but rather brain damage which prevents a person from making an intended movement. It is sometimes hard to determine whether Alzheimer's patients have trouble dressing themselves because of memory problems and the inability to grasp the logical sequence of the task or because they are exhibiting apraxia. Later in the illness, difficulties in grasping a fork, spoon, or cup, and carrying out intended movements could be due to apraxia.

Inability to recognize objects and people, agnosia, occurs.

Agnosia, an inability to recognize objects and people, is another brain disturbance in Alzheimer's disease. Agnosia is not a memory problem. Brain damage makes it impossible for information to be processed correctly. Visual information is distorted by the brain so that it is unrecognizable. The affected person may not recognize his home. At times, he may ask where his spouse is even though that spouse is sitting close by.

Number skills diminish and are lost.

The ability to do mathematic calculations is also lost with Alzheimer's disease. This is not merely a problem with memory; number skills are simply lost. Addition, subtraction, and other mathematical operations cannot be done successfully. Such problems create obstacles to successful daily living, particularly in paying bills and keeping checking accounts balanced. If the person is employed in a job that requires the use of mathematics, calculation problems may emerge before other problems are evident. This includes sales clerks as well as accountants.

Writing skills progressively erode. Writing abilities will ultimately be impaired. Initially the person may have some trouble writing paragraphs which require him to keep up with a lot of information. Gradually the ability to write sentences will erode. Words may be used incorrectly and misspelled. Eventually the person will be unable to write his name. Reading abilities may be intact longer, although grasping the meaning of what has been read disappears sooner because of memory and intellectual problems.

Another symptom of an Alzheimer's-type dementia is difficulty in drawing and copying geometric designs. Three dimensional figures are especially difficult to reproduce. The ability to draw or copy simpler figures will deteriorate as the disease progresses. Loss of these abilities may not seem significant, but the general loss of visual-spatial skills does impact daily living. Writing, reading, finding one's way in a neighborhood, or locating items in the home all involve visual-spatial abilities.

Personality changes become noticeable early. *Personality changes* occur with dementia. Usually these changes become evident after the very early stages of the illness. Some personality changes may be a reaction to unsuccessful compensations for losses in functioning; brain damage also alters the personality. With Alzheimer's disease, personality traits may become more evident and actually be accentuated. A suspicious person will probably become frankly paranoid. An individual who has always reacted strongly to little troubles will react more often and more strongly to small problems. The individual's personality will change as a result of the progressive brain damage, and the person will not seem to be himself.

Before making a diagnosis of dementia, delirium must be ruled out.

One final condition, along with the confirmation of the previously described symptoms, must be met for a diagnosis of dementia to be possible. The individual must *show clear consciousness,* which means there is no evidence that delirium is creating the symptoms. Delirium is a clouding of one's consciousness, with a decreased awareness of his immediate environment. A person who is delirious finds it difficult to shift, focus, and sustain attention to what is occurring in his environment. His perceptions of these occurrences are disturbed. Speech may be incoherent. Disorientation and memory impairment may be present, but they are caused by the delirium, not by the dementia. Persons with Alzheimer's disease may suffer delirium at times because of underlying infections or other medical problems, which make the dementia appear to have worsened.

The symptoms we have discussed represent criteria for professionals to diagnose dementia. However, before a diagnosis can be made, the cause of the dementia must be determined. There are many conditions that can cause dementia. Alzheimer's disease may be more common, but it can only be given as a probable diagnosis when all other conditions are appropriately excluded. The history of the symptoms is extremely important since some dementing conditions such as strokes occur abruptly. In others, like Parkinson's disease, dementia develops over a period of time comparable to Alzheimer's disease. Even if other potential causes for dementia have been ruled out, one must monitor the course of the condition. In some cases the progression may move very rapidly or seem to stop. Such phenomena may require some cases to be reconsidered. Severe depression may mimic dementia, but, with treatment, the dementia-like symptoms may improve.

Dementia can be caused by treatable conditions.

Some conditions that cause dementia can be treated successfully, thus reversing the dementia. We will list some of the more common of these treatable conditions. The reader should note that the conditions listed do not inevitably cause dementia, and that some conditions also can cause delirium.

Reversible Causes of Dementia Symptoms and Delirium

	Delirium	Dementia
Depression		Yes
Congestive Heart Failure	Yes	Yes
Acute Myocardial Infarct	Yes	
Renal Failure	Yes	Yes
Hypoglycemia	Yes	Yes
Hyperglycemia	Yes	Yes
Hypothyroidism	Yes	Yes
Hyperthyroidism	Yes	Yes
Pneumonia	Yes	
Diverticulitis	Yes	
Transient Ischemia	Yes	
Stroke	Yes	Yes
Subdural Hematoma	Yes	Yes
Concussion	Yes	
Neurosyphilis	Yes	Yes
Tuberculosis	Yes	Yes
Brain Tumor	Yes	Yes
Brain Abscess	Yes	Yes
Normal Pressure Hydrocephalus (abnormal flow of spinal fluid)		Yes
Fecal Impaction	Yes	
Urinary Retention	Yes	
Sensory Deprivation States (such as blindness or deafness)	Yes	Yes
Environmental Changes and Isolation	Yes	Yes
Electrolyte Abnormalities		Yes
Lifelong Alcoholism		Yes
Anemia	Yes	Yes
Chronic Lung Disease with Hypoxia	Yes	Yes
Deficiencies of Nutrients (such as vitamins B-12, folic acid, niacin)		Yes
Drug intoxication	Yes	Yes
Bladder, Urinary Tract Infection	Yes	

This list of conditions, while incomplete, illustrates the fact that a number of conditions can cause both dementia and delirium. It would be tragic for a diagnosis of Alzheimer's disease or another irreversible dementia to be given without the proper physical examination, laboratory, and other diagnostic tests being completed. Such tests may reveal that a person has a treatable condition. The importance of the appropriate medical personnel being involved in some part of the evaluation of dementia cannot be stressed enough.

Along with these treatable conditions, other irreversible dementias (those that cannot be treated) must be considered. Alzheimer's disease is the most common irreversible dementia, followed by multi-infarct dementia, which is caused by multiple strokes. About 50 percent of all dementias of the elderly are caused by Alzheimer's disease; 20 percent to 25 percent are caused by multi-infarct disease, and another 20 percent of dementias are caused by a combination of these two conditions. Other conditions account for less than 10 percent of dementias. The following list illustrates some of these irreversible dementias. We will list only the more commonly known conditions. Of course, some of these are still quite rare, for example, Creutzfeldt-Jakob disease and Pick's disease. General Paresis, which is a form of central nervous system syphilis, is becoming rare with the successful treatment of syphilis.

Irreversible Dementias

Alzheimer's Disease
Pick's Disease
Multi-Infarct Dementia
Creutzfeldt-Jakob Disease
Kuru
General Paresis
Parkinson's Disease
Huntington's Disease
Wilson's Disease

Multi-infarct dementia must be ruled out before making a diagnosis of Alzheimer's.

Multi-infarct dementia is the second leading cause of dementia and must be ruled out when Alzheimer's disease is suspected. There is also a group of psychiatric disorders that can mimic dementia; these disorders, because they are not true dementias, are called pseudodementias. Ordinarily, depression is considered as a pseudodementia when it is severe enough to create symptoms of dementia. In addition, schizophrenia can create symptoms suggestive of dementia. Without adequate personal history, it may be difficult to determine whether symptoms are caused by the thought disorder or dementia. We will discuss multi-infarct dementia in some detail, since it is likely to be considered a potential cause of dementia in initial evaluations. (Depression, another likely candidate related to dementia, is discussed at length in Chapter 3.)

Cumulative effects of several strokes can create dementia. Most people are familiar with strokes, which cause varying degrees of damage to the brain. The cumulative effects of multiple strokes create dementia by damaging multiple areas of the brain. A single stroke or "infarct" will not usually cause dementia, even though initially this may appear to be the case. However, after the stroke, a person will usually move toward some degree of recovery. With some patients recovery may be partial, but with many recovery can be fairly complete, leaving no significant effects on everyday functioning.

Strokes are caused by blockages in blood vessels or arteries. The types and severity of strokes vary. Some strokes are caused by blockage of large- or medium-sized blood vessels. Blockage of a large artery can produce massive brain damage, impairing intellectual abilities, voluntary movements, and speech. The brain damage associated with blockage of blood vessels or small arteries may not be so apparent. For instance, the effects of such strokes on intellectual functioning or voluntary movement are so subtle they may not be recognized. Subsequent strokes could occur, involving other small arteries. The cumulative damage of these multiple strokes likely would produce an emerging picture of dementia. When the cumulative effects of small strokes cannot be adequately observed and monitored, it is more difficult to determine whether the dementia is due to multiple small strokes or whether the deterioration of brain functioning is attributable to a primary dementia like Alzheimer's disease.

A single stroke usually results in fairly specific symptoms which do not meet all the criteria for a diagnosis of dementia. Some of the problems caused by strokes include paralysis and restriction of voluntary movement; speech difficulties, ranging from the inability to form words clearly to problems using and comprehending words correctly (expressive and receptive aphasia); emotional instability (moods change rapidly); and impairment of memory or intellectual abilities. When symptoms are pronounced, they will also appear abruptly. If more than one stroke occurs, the deficits will appear to follow a stepwise deteriorating course. One more stroke will occur. Then the affected person will show some progress and improve. If another stroke occurs, other deficits will be evident. Some recovery will take place, but each time another stroke occurs, the overall level of abilities will deteriorate another step. The deficits will not involve all functions of the person initially, but subsequent strokes will create dementia, a multi-infarct dementia.

One kind of stroke is difficult to differentiate from Alzheimer's. The results of one type of stroke are very difficult to differentiate from Alzheimer's disease. Called an "angular gyrus syndrome," this kind of stroke involves the brain area supplied with blood and nutrients by the middle cerebral artery (Cummings and Benson 1983). Predisposing medical factors are hypertension or cardiac disease. Aphasia, writing difficulties, calculation deficits, disorientation of right-left sides, and memory problems (actually word-finding difficulties) are some of the symptoms of this kind of stroke. The stroke patient may be apologetic about and frustrated with his language performance; however, the Alzheimer's patient will be unaware of such problems and be more difficult to involve in conversation (Cummings and Benson 1983).

A CAT scan can usually help identify larger stroke damage to the brain. However, small strokes cannot always be detected, which can be the case with the angular gyrus syndrome; often the damaged area is very small.

Multi-infarct dementia must be ruled out before a group of

symptoms can indicate an Alzheimer's-type dementia. Sometimes the professionals involved in the evaluation process may have to clearly identify differences in symptoms to make a distinction between Alzheimer's disease and multi-infarct dementia. Laboratory tests, medical history, or even a CAT scan cannot always be helpful in making that distinction.

Even though strokes cause an abrupt appearance of symptoms, a stroke victim may not be aware of the subtle changes caused by a small stroke. Families may be unable to identify such changes in behavior, or they may attribute them to other causes. Strokes are usually painless. They may even occur while the person is sleeping. Early symptoms resulting from some strokes can include dizziness, headaches, and decreased physical and mental vigor. There may be vague physical complaints. Despite the fact strokes can occur suddenly, the onset can be gradual. Such a presentation can be easily confused with Alzheimer's disease. Many times the onset of a stroke is signaled by confusion.

Strokes can have other features that do not necessarily suggest brain damage. The affected individual may demonstrate poor judgment and insight at times. Delirium may occur, and family members may observe hallucinations. Emotional changes may be prevalent. The person who has had a stroke may not exhibit tact or sensitivity in social situations. His concern for others can diminish, and the narrowing of interests in other people and things can lead to increasing self-preoccupation. Depression is not an uncommon consequence of strokes.

Medical conditions create risk for strokes. There are numbers of medical conditions that create risk for strokes. Hypertension, diabetes, and cardiac disease are associated with strokes and multi-infarct dementia. Since strokes are a major cause of death, the suspicion of a stroke should never be treated lightly. If a stroke has occurred, aggressive medical treatment may prevent subsequent strokes, which could lead to a multi-infarct dementia. Additionally, persons known to have Alzheimer's disease can suffer strokes. This possibility is very real; in fact from 20 percent to 25 percent of dementias are caused by a combination of Alzheimer's disease and multi-infarct disease. When it is possible to prevent a stroke or subsequent strokes in an Alzheimer's patient, compounded disabilities can be avoided.

Phases of Alzheimer's Disease

Rate of progressive deterioration varies.

Many illnesses follow stages of development and recovery. With Alzheimer's, however, there is no recovery; the slow, progressive course leads to further deterioration of behavior and abilities. For some victims, particularly those under 60, the stages move rapidly, and the illness results in death within three to five years. When the onset begins at a later age, however, the disease may progress slowly for ten years or more.

Understanding of the illness helps adjustment.

Both the person who is in the early stages of Alzheimer's and his family naturally want to know what to expect as the illness progresses. An understanding of what is to come allows the family to prepare for future stages, to ease the victim's adjustment, and to gradually accept the disease's effect on the whole family.

Understanding stages helps both families and professionals.

The stages of the disease discussed in this chapter are essentially those developed by Dr. Barry Reisberg, Associate Professor of Psychiatry at New York University Medical Center. A general knowledge of these stages can help both families and professionals to do the following:

- Accurately assess and diagnose the condition
- Identify symptoms and follow their progression as the illness develops
- Determine the rate at which the illness is developing
- Have realistic expectations of the patient's capabilities

- Evaluate the adjustment of both family and patient
- Assist family with utilization of appropriate resources.

Manifestations of deficits are dependent upon many factors. Not all Alzheimer's conditions will exactly follow the gradual breakdown indicated in the discussion of stages which follows. There are individual variations that can be attributed to numerous factors: the person's intelligence and abilities before the illness, his personality and basic ways of coping with problems, other health problems, marital relationship, and degree of environmental support.

Stage I: Early Confusional Phase

Forgetfulness becomes a problem. During the beginning stages of Alzheimer's, the patient may seem merely forgetful. As his memory problems worsen, however, the patient's social and occupational skills will begin to diminish noticeably. Although he will usually deny his growing memory problems and successfully compensate at times, he will not be able to catch all of his mistakes.

Confusion and slower responses affect driving. In the early stages, it becomes harder for the person to deal with change and new things. If he travels to an unfamiliar area, he may become lost and confused. However, he probably can still travel familiar routes alone. In traffic, he will be slower to react as his powers of concentration and memory decrease.

Early problems with social conversation During this phase, the person may have trouble finding the right words to communicate his thoughts. Problems in recalling the names of new people and recent conversations may be increasingly apparent. Similarly, he may retain little information from books, magazines, or television shows.

Personality changes appear. The person will begin to lose his spontaneity and sparkle. Socially speaking, he will be slower and less discriminating in what he says and does. His lessened initiative, energy, and drive will be noticeable. He will become more easily upset, anxious, and angry as a result of the uncertainties created by his memory problems. This anxiety, most evident when the person is in demanding social or work-related situations, may cause him to completely avoid unfamiliar or difficult situations.

Denial conceals recognition of early problems. Despite a person's degree of impairment during this early stage, his family may be aware of only a few specific problems. The individual will be using his remaining strengths to cover for his deficits. This denial often leads family members to discount the severity of the person's problems. A person going through the first stages of Alzheimer's disease seems distressed, but the reasons are often a mystery to those closest to him.

Early emotional symptoms are brought to the attention of mental health professionals. At this point, because the symptoms seem to be emotional rather than physical, psychiatrists and other mental health professionals are most likely to be called upon for diagnosis and treatment. Medications might be considered to manage the emotional symptoms. It is important to note that not all persons who exhibit characteristics of the first stage of Alzheimer's disease actually have Alzheimer's. However, if the symptoms of Alzheimer's are present, a diagnosis should be sought, even though it may be distressing to face the full implications of the person's behavior. A victim of Alzheimer's will change gradually but dramatically, and it is both unfair and unrealistic to go on treating the person exactly as in the past.

The disease process results in changes in abilities and actions. It is critical to understand that the Alzheimer's victim's problems are not caused by mere laziness, carelessness, or momentary irrational behavior. The disease is the culprit, and the caregiver must begin to prepare himself for the worsening of problems as the victim slowly declines.

Stage II: Late Confusional Phase

Memory problems are more evident.
As Alzheimer's disease progresses, problems with memory become more evident and somewhat more pervasive. For example, the person's retention of current events declines. He will easily lose the thread of a story and have noticeable difficulties in following conversations. His responses will fail to correspond to the situation. Likewise, his memory of personal history may become foggy.

Decision making and financial management deteriorate.
Making plans or decisions becomes extremely difficult for the person and equally as frustrating for the family. Family members may feel the need to help their relative with his finances and other important responsibilities as it becomes obvious that he is not handling them well.

The denial of problem makes the family's job more difficult.
The affected relative may not welcome assistance. He still may be denying his problems and may see any assistance as interference. The caregiver may see the victim's refusal to admit both his problems and his need for help as impaired judgment. These differences in perception can begin to generate even more conflict within the family. In addition, the victim may choose to avoid social situations altogether as they become too difficult to handle.

Driving becomes riskier.
The person's driving also becomes a source of concern. At this stage, the Alzheimer's patient probably can travel familiar routes with reasonable safety. However, he is vulnerable to mistakes and improper responses to unforeseen situations. He may overreact or not react at all to potentially dangerous traffic conditions. The family should seriously consider curtailing or eliminating driving opportunities.

Orientation in time and place is affected. Some aspects of the person's memory—his orientation to time, place, and person—may still be intact at this stage. However, his difficulties in concentrating may make it difficult to recall these things or to recall the events of the past few minutes or the past week. On the other hand, memories of the distant past can be surprisingly clear and accurate. He may speak more often about past events and avoid conversations about current events.

Supervision means supportive assistance. The Alzheimer's victim will need some supervision and daily support during this stage. Although he is not disabled in all aspects of his life, he will need help in more complex areas such as handling his finances and paying his bills. The mixture of stress and detailed organization necessary to file income tax reports, balance a checkbook, and pay bills may be more than he can handle.

The victim becomes self-absorbed and depressed. As the victim sees his capabilities slipping away, he is likely to become increasingly self-absorbed and insensitive to the feelings of others. Often, the victim sinks into depression, making his situation even worse. The caregiver, trying to assist a loved one with problems he denies having, can easily feel rejected and unappreciated.

Stage III: Early Dementia

Dependency increases the caregiver's load. By this time, the Alzheimer's victim has become quite dependent on others for his care. That dependency increases the caregiver's sense of responsibility for meeting all of the person's needs and keeping him safe from harm. It is difficult for someone who is not involved in the actual care to understand how much must be done daily. In fact, other family members may fail to support the primary caregiver because they cannot envision how strenuous the mental and physical demands of daily caregiving are. A person in the early dementia phase requires:

- Help in initiating most activities
- Someone to help him "think"
- "Hands-on" care as his dependencies increase
- Help in expressing his needs.

The victim should not drive. A person who is exhibiting symptoms of early dementia is a hazardous driver. For example, he may increase his speed or drive through stop signs unknowingly. Likewise, stressful situations encountered while driving can dramatically affect his judgment. Family members therefore must take it upon themselves to ensure that the patient does not drive.

Memory gaps trigger insecurity and defensive behavior. Even though his problems are obvious to everyone around, the patient may continue to deny and shield his mistakes. In conversations he may fabricate information that seems irrelevant or absurd. Actually, he is valiantly trying to fill in information gaps created by memory loss. The patient is trying to pull together pieces of his own reality in order to maintain a meaningful life.

As his memory deteriorates, a heightened sense of insecurity can develop into suspicion and paranoia. Judgment and reasoning deteriorate further. His suspiciousness may be accompanied by anger, even when a family member tries to prove his accusations or suspicions are unfounded. Agitated behavior may develop.

Emotional reactions become more prominent. The patient's emotional instability comes from a mixture of psychological, social, and neurological sources. During this stage, the Alzheimer's patient may have periodic crying spells and abrupt mood changes, with or without obvious causes. Such instability can be frightening and aggravating to families. Soothing, calming approaches that convey support and understanding are good responses on the caregiver's part.

Memory deficits fluctuate. Fluctuations in memory on an almost moment-to-moment basis are not uncommon in Stage III. Caregivers should realize that such fluctuations are a normal part of the disease, making the best of those days when their relative seems better, and avoiding despondency when he seems worse.

Logical, sequential reasoning and actions diminish. The victim's ability to recall the correct sequences of behavior and tasks becomes seriously impaired. This inability may show up in areas such as dressing or grooming, where he may complete only part of the task.

Independence encouraged Usually, he can continue to perform part of his daily routine with help. It is easy, however, to increase his dependency unnecessarily by assuming certain things are too intricate for him to complete. For example, by Stage III he will need help in selecting properly matched and appropriate clothing, but this does not mean he cannot still dress himself. Some persons with Alzheimer's will want to wear the same clothes every day, without changing or washing them. Although this kind of behavior will tempt caregivers to take over the entire task, the patient should be encouraged to care for himself as long as possible.

Simple decisions become overwhelming. During early dementia, a person will have difficulty making even simple decisions concerning eating or dressing. But the caregiver still can offer simple alternatives that require a yes or no response. It may be helpful to suggest a choice of two necessary alternatives, such as bathing or picking up the dirty clothes. This increases the chance that the patient will undertake at least one desirable course of action.

Social withdrawal is accompanied by impaired thinking capacity. The affected person can be expected to withdraw from both social and task-oriented activities. His decreasing thinking and reasoning abilities will make him less flexible and able to adjust to stressful situations. If he is pushed, he will become both overly anxious and angry; if he is pushed too often, he will refuse to do even necessary stressful activities. Nonetheless, he may still enjoy some social situations. For example, going to church or the movies may still be fairly undemanding, while visiting with long-time friends may be overwhelming.

Caregivers require support. At this point, caregivers need considerable emotional support and relief from their full-time responsibilities. Family members, friends, and neighbors can provide both the support and the relief the primary caregiver needs, whether it is by sitting with the relative, doing chores, or visiting. Caregivers should carefully monitor their own ability to handle the demands placed upon them, and they should not hesitate to ask for help as needed.

Stage IV: Middle Dementia

The victim reacts more severely to loss of abilities. Major changes occur as the disease progresses from early to middle dementia, and the involvement of caregivers increases considerably. Throughout the illness, the patient may have been fairly successful in using denial to protect himself from the realization that his mind is slipping away. However, denial is becoming a less effective protector. Withdrawal is being replaced by tendencies toward agitation, paranoia, and delusions. The need for security cannot be satisfied by the victim's mind. At this point, the environment can meet this need through structure, routine, and caring.

Delusions Delusions often reflect fears of loss and imagined threats in the external world. Spouses may be accused of being unfaithful. Neighbors and friends may be blamed for unbelievable things.

Sleep distur-
bances and
hallucinations

During this phase, the patient's sleep is more often disrupted and erratic. He may be awakened by hallucinations or delusional fears that make it almost impossible to sleep, and he may begin to wander at night.

Repetitive
behavior

A number of emotional changes appear during the middle dementia stage. They may include compulsive symptoms such as pulling clothes out of drawers and replacing them over and over. The person may not be able to hold onto his thoughts long enough to complete a course of action. Obsessive thoughts or repetitive ideas and concerns may be more evident in some persons.

Movement and
coordination
difficulties

The victim's problems with movement and coordination may become more obvious now and interfere markedly with his performance. He will develop difficulties with walking and with the purposeful, coordinated movements required for dressing, eating, brushing his teeth, and so forth. Eating difficulties may contribute to weight loss; alternatively, excessive eating may become a problem.

Help with daily
activities is
essential.

At this point, the Alzheimer's victim requires assistance with most activities of daily living. The caregiver must carefully and sensitively adjust his social and behavioral expectations of the patient downward. The individual must not be placed in situations that could lead to emotional overload; he could overreact in violent and frightening ways.

Sources of vio-
lent behavior

Much of the violent behavior of persons with Alzheimer's disease is triggered by excessive environmental demands. The person is unable to comprehend what behavior is expected of him and may respond inappropriately. Pressure to respond to situations promptly further accentuates inappropriate responses. Too many choices or options can precipitate more anxiety and agitation or may lead to further withdrawal.

Bathing problems emerge. The middle dementia stage brings a real fear of bathing. This fear is often misinterpreted by caregivers as simple stubbornness and uncooperativeness. But actually, the person's fear of bathing is related to reasonable concerns. The patient forgets how to adjust water temperature and how to use the soap and washcloth. His impaired coordination creates difficulties in getting in and out of the tub, and he may fear falling. In addition, the patient has lost his sense of the social importance of personal hygiene. To reduce conflict over bathing, the caregiver may substitute towel washing for a tub bath or reduce the frequency of bathing. Sometimes the patient may accept a hot bath as a way to relieve tensions, especially when it is combined with a soothing body massage.

Loss of touch with events and experiences Persons in middle dementia are generally unaware of their surroundings, the time of year, the year itself, and other indications of time and place. Memory abilities deteriorate to a fragmentary knowledge of home address and whereabouts. Getting lost becomes almost inevitable and is a real worry for caregivers. The patient may be able to distinguish strangers from familiar persons, but often he cannot identify the person on whom he is most dependent, his spouse. He will usually know his own name and have some sketchy recall of his past, but he is largely unaware of all recent events and experiences. He may give pieces of information which have no clear meaning. For the victim of Alzheimer's, the world has become frightening and largely unmanageable. The loss of cognitive, memory, and perceptual abilities prevents him from organizing the pieces of his life into a meaningful whole.

Caregiving becomes lonelier and more isolating. At this stage, caregiving takes up most of the day and night, yet the caregiver receives little or no recognition from the patient. Kindness is rarely seen, unless it is read into some small action or gesture. This is extremely difficult for many caregivers to accept, since they naturally seek gratitude and approval from their relative.

If the caregiver has assumed solitary care for the victim, he is likely to become severely isolated, both physically and socially. Friends no longer visit, and community activities are restricted. The greatest isolation is created by the inability of the victim to relate to the caregiver spouse. All decisions fall on his shoulders. There are no rewards and appreciation for the caregiving, unless the caregiver finds ways to affirm himself and compensate for the emotional isolation and separation.

Caregiver must hire help or place the victim in an institution. By this stage, the emotional burdens of caregiving force those involved to make difficult decisions about whether to hire in-home help or possibly place the person in an institution. In Stage IV, hiring full-time assistance is the ideal situation for caregivers. However, it is costly to hire experienced full-time help; thus part-time help may be the best alternative. But the primary caregiver must have some relief from the consuming tasks of direct care and supervision. In addition, the patient may need some form of psychiatric or other professional mental health assistance.

Caregivers need support groups. Even with help, the caregiver's role may become so demanding as to totally overwhelm his life. The patient's sleeping problems are likely to disrupt the caregiver's sleep; his agitation makes management more perplexing and tiring; his delusional beliefs are painful and frightening. A family support group can help. The caregiver may also feel a need for individual counseling and assistance in securing other supportive resources.

The caregiver should call upon the whole family for help and support as needed. Major decisions regarding other arrangements for the patient's final weeks, months, or years are forthcoming, and few caregivers should be making such decisions without some degree of family input and support.

When family members do not support the most appropriate course of action, the primary caregiver must be reassured by others that he is making the correct decisions. Conflicts may develop because relatives do not understand the implications of the illness and the daily strains of caregiving.

Stage V: Late Dementia

Such phrases as "a long good-bye" or an "unending death" have been used to describe the disease's final stage. Caregivers must give so much for so small a response that often all the questions of life seem to be best summed up in one word—"WHY?"

Recognize limitations of caregiving. Decisions now must be made without the loved one's nod of approval. Notions of what is best or what he would have wanted compete with the fact that one must decide alone. As narrow as the victim's life has become, it is still valuable to the family, and it is hard to say good-bye. Nonetheless, one hopes to see the suffering end. Although the caregiver may want to keep his loved one at home, an institution may be the only realistic alternative when he can no longer provide full-time care.

Denial may continue to protect the victim from the emotional impact of the illness. He may still be able to smile, to laugh, and to appear to enjoy life at times.

There is less of everything. The emotional experience of life can go on even though the words have been lost. Behaviorally, the person is as likely to be amenable as he is to be difficult. The need for tranquilizers lessens because his behavior has become more easily managed.

His motor abilities will continue to deteriorate and eventually his ability to walk, sit, and smile will be lost, as well as his control of bladder and colon functions. The loss may be uneven: a person who is still walking may be found on the floor or caught as he falls because he suddenly has forgotten how to walk. Such cases may require medical attention to ensure that a stroke or transient ischemic attack (condition in which blood supply to the brain is temporarily interrupted) has not occurred.

Addressing movement problems

It is important to help the Alzheimer's victim to walk as long as he is able. He will not be able to use a walker, since he has lost his coordination, but guardrails and other supports can help. In addition, rearranging furniture to provide support and eliminating barriers (such as loose rugs) will help the individual in his walking. The use of geriatric chairs and other confining devices should be avoided as much as possible; such confinement increases agitation and restlessness.

Eating difficulties

During this final stage, the patient will eventually lose the ability to chew and swallow food. The caregiver may have to cut the food into small pieces or prepare an almost totally soft diet. If the patient refuses to eat, other methods of feeding must be considered.

Need more structured, highly supervised care

As brain activity becomes severely disturbed, the patient is increasingly vulnerable to seizures as well as aspiration, pneumonia, infection, and other illnesses. He will need assistance in eating, since choking, blockage, or other problems in breathing and swallowing can occur. Respiratory problems can worsen through decreased activity, particularly when the person becomes bedridden.

The final reconciliation

Stupor occurs in this terminal stage and leads finally to coma and death. Throughout the illness, the caregiver has had to meet one challenge after another in caring for his loved one. Human contact has made a real difference to the Alzheimer's victim. Such contact is still important, even if the person is seemingly unable to respond. Patience and kindness, though they require great strength, are necessary. A touch, a loving voice, and the presence of a loved one help keep a person physically and emotionally alive, even when he can no longer reach out to anyone.

3

DEPRESSION AND ALZHEIMER'S

Depression is a serious psychiatric condition. Although we commonly use the term "depressed" to describe someone who is feeling down or out-of-sorts, severe depression is actually a serious psychiatric condition. Unlike the temporary moodiness that is normal to daily life, clinical depression is not a condition that one recovers from easily, although the condition can be cured. Because depression often accompanies Alzheimer's disease, it is important that caregivers learn to recognize the condition and seek treatment for symptoms.

Symptoms of depression Depression is a prolonged disturbance of mood that colors a person's whole inner perception of the world. She feels down in the dumps, unworthy, and may feel that life is not worth living. The symptoms of depression include feelings of sadness and emptiness, withdrawal from others, self-neglect, sleeping problems, and many other emotional and physical signs, which are listed in more detail later in this chapter. Because many of these same symptoms also accompany Alzheimer's disease, it is easy for depression to go unrecognized and untreated in an Alzheimer's patient.

Professional help should be sought. If caregivers suspect that their loved one is seriously depressed, they should not hesitate to seek psychiatric treatment, which can be quite beneficial. In a few cases, a patient suffering from depression may even have been diagnosed mistakenly as having Alzheimer's. It is therefore important that a check for depression be made as part of the diagnostic work-up for all patients suffering from an Alzheimer's-type dementia.

Depression is more likely in the early stages. A person with Alzheimer's is most likely to suffer from severe depression during the earlier stages of the illness, when she still has the faculties to comprehend the full implications of the disease. The disturbing changes she is experiencing naturally lead her to become depressed about the future, but her depression in turn may intensify the effects of the disease.

Risk factors for depression Persons who have previously suffered from depression are at a particular risk of becoming depressed in the face of Alzheimer's. Also at risk are highly achievement-oriented and perfectionist personalities. Difficult social and family situations can trigger depression, particularly when the victim lacks any source of emotional support. In other cases depression may be brought on simply by reduced self-esteem or loss of income caused by Alzheimer's. Denial of this illness may not be sufficient protection from what is happening.

Symptoms of depression are hard to recognize in an Alzheimer's victim. The symptoms of depression can be hard to isolate and recognize when Alzheimer's is present although they should be evident to a mental health professional. Often a close evaluation is required to determine whether Alzheimer's or depression or both are causing a particular behavior. For example, the urge to withdraw from social situations could indicate either condition, but reasons may be different.

Depression characterized by a number of symptoms Like dementia, depression is characterized by a cluster of symptoms. Although none of these symptoms is necessarily significant alone, when they exist in combination for an extended period of time, a severe depression may be indicated.

Physical symptoms of depression   Numerous physical complaints that cannot be explained by any known medical problem may indicate depression. Such physical symptoms include:

- Weakness, unexplained fatigue, dizzy spells, low energy
- Gastrointestinal problems such as pain, indigestion, constipation
- Urinary disturbances
- Changes in eating habits, appetite, and weight
- Loss of sexual desire
- Sleeping disturbances, including awakening during the night or early morning awakening
- Slowed movement or more agitated movement
- Slowed speech; softened, lowered, or monotone voice; incomplete responses.

Psychological symptoms of depression   Depression also brings on a whole range of psychological symptoms. These may include:

- Tension, anxiety, and irritability
- Loss of initiative and interest
- Indecisiveness and ambivalence
- Inability to take pleasure in favorite activities
- Apathy, boredom, indifference, and resisting activity
- Doing little or nothing
- Loss of interest in grooming and personal care
- Poor attention and concentration
- Extreme sensitivity to problems with memory
- Excessive complaints and worries
- Tendency to cry and get upset over little things.

Guilt, suicidal ideas, sense of inadequacy, and hopelessness   Other common symptoms associated with depression include expressions of guilt and concern about making up for perceived wrongs done to others or omissions of responsibilities toward family and friends. Preoccupations with death and suicidal ideas or the desire to die occur in more serious depression. In earlier stages of Alzheimer's, the depressed person's suicidal ideas must be taken particularly seriously. Feelings of failure, inadequacy, helplessness, and powerlessness all characterize the low self-evaluation of a depressed person. An underlying dementia further stimulates and reinforces such views. Negative expectations, self-blame, and self-criticism can reinforce each other to create a downward emotional spiral.

Seek professional help for depression.

Many depressed persons deny some of the emotional symptoms of the illness or have difficulty reporting them. Should symptoms characteristic of depression be noted during the progression of Alzheimer's, caregivers need to seek professional help. Some of these symptoms could be suggestive of an ongoing grief process, but this should be evaluated by a professional familiar with depression. Treatment of depression is important, for it can improve both the person's outlook and functioning.

Caregivers also suffer from depression.

Caregivers may recognize some of the symptoms described here developing in themselves. Though these may be brought on by grief or stress rather than clinical depression, caregivers who experience the symptoms of depression should consult a mental health professional. Caring for an Alzheimer's patient is difficult enough without the added burden of a severe depression.

A case example: The impact depression has in Alzheimer's disease.

Harry Sims, a 54-year-old male, came to our center one day with his wife Julie who was 47 years old. Recently, Harry had learned he had Alzheimer's disease. It had been diagnosed at a major medical center. He made light of his diagnosis because his principal concern was his wife's adjustment to the illness. They had only been married for five years and her 13-year-old son lived in the household. Harry had a business of his own.

Julie had helped with the business, but her husband had always been in total control of everything he did. He was also a perfectionist, and her work had never been remotely acceptable to him. His strong personality was a definite contrast to her own. She was reserved and reticent. Julie had serious doubts about her abilities, and her self-esteem was quite low. Her husband's illness was frightening to her.

She was equally apprehensive about their financial future. She questioned how long Harry could continue to handle the business. His solution to this was to have her run the business or find someone else that he could trust to run it with his assistance. Harry had very high expectations of his wife, and he would put great pressure on any other person who became responsible for the business. It was more significant that Harry placed even greater pressure on himself.

Mr. Sims' concerns about his wife's adjustment to the illness translated into his concerns about the family business. His lack of confidence in his wife heightened his insecurity about this matter. He seemed to project any of his shortcomings onto his wife. This had worsened over the past year and created considerable tension between the couple. Another sore point concerned Julie's son. He could not walk the line for his stepfather, and the two battled constantly. This was a matter of great distress for Julie who seemed to be stuck in the middle.

Over a period of several weeks the couple came for counseling. They were able to make some improvements. Julie, particularly, began to appreciate what was beginning to happen to her husband. Nevertheless, tensions continued to build. Harry became progressively more hostile and verbally aggressive. They stayed in separate parts of their home and no longer had meals together. The conflict between Harry and his stepson escalated. Over one weekend, tempers flared, and the situation exploded; the wife and her son left the house and stayed with friends.

On Monday of the following week they came to our center in separate cars. Our psychiatrist saw both, and medication was given on a trial basis to reduce Harry's extreme agitation and hostile behavior. After two weeks, it appeared the situation had improved somewhat. This was partly attributable to the fact that Julie's son had gone to live with a brother and his family.

Julie was having as difficult a time as Harry in her own way. When she and Harry were seen together, it was clear that she was suffering from clinical depression. Her appetite was poor, and she was not sleeping well at night. Her ability to concentrate and remember was affected. She experienced extreme anxiety and was apprehensive of her husband much of the time. Her energy level was very low, and fatigue had become a constant complaint. Stomach distress was a major physical complaint. Her low self-esteem was even lower and she had helpless and hopeless feelings. It was terrible to consider the future. She was given an antidepressant medication.

Considerable improvement was noted when she and her husband came again in two weeks. Their relationship had improved slightly. She was having more contact with her few friends. This had been a recommendation because she was isolated. Harry had few friends himself and had initially controlled her contact with the few friends they did have. They lived 10 miles outside a small rural city, which accentuated the sense of isolation and loneliness that Julie experienced.

Several factors were considered before Harry and Julie returned for their next appointment. First, Harry had a very high need for control which he was losing. His wife had become a liability as his own denial of the illness failed to protect him. He had often stated that he could handle the Alzheimer's disease. It became clear that his attempts to get help for his wife were actually attempts to get help for himself. The security of remaining life was dependent upon someone else. Before, Harry had not been able to depend upon or trust anyone.

Harry had never demonstrated any of the memory impairment typical of Alzheimer's disease. Few people would have believed that he could have Alzheimer's disease. The major effect of the illness was on his speech. His speech was pressured and circumlocutory. He tended to repeat himself a little. There was a problem in expressing ideas clearly, and Harry admitted he had trouble getting his thoughts together. Nevertheless, he demonstrated skillful compensations for any underlying deficits. The agitation and low tolerance for frustration created the biggest problem in his business. He got too easily upset with his customers and became overwhelmed more easily by work demand.

There was reasonable doubt in some minds about whether he actually had Alzheimer's disease, but the medical center had been thorough in its evaluation. We began to suspect that he was suffering from depression. He complained some about fatigue and concentration, both of which are not uncommon in Alzheimer's disease. However, Harry usually denied having any significant problems with memory. There were many more somatic complaints. He had a distracting ringing in his ears and experienced some pain in his legs. He had stomach distress and complained of headaches. Tension, anxiety, and agitation were quite evident.

Harry's personality style provided other clues. He had some paranoid tendencies that were consistent with the controlling, compulsive traits. It was significant that he had few friends and did not form relationships easily. In fact, he was somewhat aloof and seldom spoke in a language of feelings. This all led to the conclusion that we were dealing with a masked depression that was associated with agitation. It was somatically characterized.

An antidepressant medication was prescribed, and the medication for the agitation was discontinued. Careful monitoring of the medication revealed no significant side effects. The only complaint was a dry mouth. A remarkable change was observed in a very short time. In two weeks this husband and wife reported that their relationship was better than it had ever been. As treatment continued, Harry began to voice the nightmare he had been living before the antidepressant was given. His fears about the illness surfaced, and we were able to deal with these feelings. He also showed that he was aware of how destructive his role in the family had become. He swallowed a great deal of pride to indicate that he had been wrong about some things, including mistakes with his stepson.

Harry and Julie began to find pleasure and enjoyment in their lives again. Harry was more accepting of his wife and other people. They were able to move to a smaller rent house they owned in town. This afforded them the opportunity to have more social contact. Harry was aware that the medication actually helped clear his thinking some. All of the somatic complaints were gone within the first two weeks.

This story began seven months ago. Harry exhibits some slight deterioration (visual-spatial problems, memory, and abstract reasoning), but some major issues are resolved. The business is presently being operated by him and his wife. His expectations are more realistic. The other critical change makes an even greater difference. The relationship with Julie's son has been reestablished, and the couple has more involvement with their respective families.

Our example above illustrates several points. First, it may be quite difficult to distinguish depression from Alzheimer's disease, particularly in some individuals and situations. Secondly, both the suspected Alzheimer's patient and caregiver spouse can be depressed. The nature of their respective coping styles can aggravate the situation even more. Depression itself is strengthened. Finally, old conflicts that have been largely unresolved can surface in such stressful caregiving situations. The needs and problems of all family members must be considered in treatment.

Recognizing and treating depression with Alzheimer's disease is a very significant intervention. Caregivers may be prone to develop depression or serious reactions to continuous stress. For this reason professionals must carefully consider how family caregivers are coping with the physical, emotional, and social aspects of the disease. Support and learning new ways to deal effectively with the demands of caregiving can be helpful, but depression may require other treatment approaches such as antidepressant medications.

4

POSSIBLE CAUSES OF ALZHEIMER'S DISEASE

Background to research Research into Alzheimer's disease has produced several schools of thought about possible causes of the disease. Some researchers theorize a single cause; others suspect that the disease results from the interaction of several different contributing factors. These might include a genetic predisposition, outside factors such as a virus, imbalances in the body such as a disorder of the immune system, and psychosocial factors such as depression, environment, stress reactions, and so forth.

Of the many causes suspected, the only one generally regarded as a certain factor, in at least some individuals, is genetic predisposition. Because this genetic factor is the most firmly established, we will discuss it in some depth. Other less well-proven theories that will be discussed briefly are those concerning slow viruses, immune-system imbalances, and excess aluminum.

It also appears highly likely that certain psychosocial factors can contribute to when Alzheimer's disease develops and the apparent severity of its symptoms. We therefore will look at the possible relevancy for Alzheimer's of such psychosocial factors as environment, psychiatric history, social and sensory deprivation, and one's sense of support and control.

What does not cause Alzheimer's A word also seems in order about what does NOT cause Alzheimer's disease. It is not caused by simple old age, hardening of the arteries, or stroke. Most importantly, it is not caused by the person's character or behavior. "Bad" or "lazy" people do not develop Alzheimer's disease any more often than "good" people. No one has ever "deserved" to get Alzheimer's disease. Although caregivers and others struggling to understand the inexplicable may be tempted to create such explanations, perhaps subconsciously, it can only make a difficult situation unnecessarily harder to imagine that the victim or anyone else is to blame for the disease. The seemingly "crazy" behavior of an Alzheimer's victim is brought about by very real physical and chemical changes in the brain (see Chapter 11) over which the person can have no control. Let us hope the true causes of these changes and of the disease itself can be identified soon.

The Genetic Theory

Genetic factors play a role in Alzheimer's disease.

Research has determined that genetic factors do play a role in Alzheimer's disease. To date, however, the disease has not been shown to widely correspond to known patterns of inheritance. Only a handful of families known to research (just over fifty) show a classic heredity pattern for Alzheimer's disease—what is known as "autosomal-dominant inheritance." In one well-regarded study of relatives of 125 Alzheimer's patients, some genetic predisposition toward the disease did appear, but the researchers concluded that both a genetic factor and another factor or factors must be involved (Heston et al. 1981).

Genetic factors combine with unidentified factors to cause Alzheimer's disease.

Genetic markers for a familial form of Alzheimer's have been identified. However, it appears that some people with genetic markers for Alzheimer's do not get the disease, while others with no apparent genetic predisposition are stricken. Many researchers thus theorize that genetic factors may combine with other factors to produce the disease in certain individuals.

Research into the genetic basis of the disease has included studies comparing the features of familial versus nonfamilial Alzheimer's, twin pairs with and without Alzheimer's, and irregularities in the chromosomes in Alzheimer's victims. The study on twins concluded that outside factors seem to determine when a person with genetic risk will actually get the disease (Nee et al. 1983).

A genetic defect is responsible for familial Alzheimer's. Genetic factors are known to play a part in other brain diseases and disorders, including Down's syndrome, which shares several features in common with Alzheimer's disease. Several studies have focused on this association. One in particular tested the theory that a gene on chromosome 21 (there are extra copies of chromosome 21 in Down's syndrome victims) may be responsible for Alzheimer's disease (St. George-Hyslop, Tanzi, et al. 1987). This study produced the first clear evidence that a genetic defect (an abnormal gene) on chromosome 21 is in fact responsible for the autosomal-dominant pattern of inheritance seen in certain families.

Amyloid is related to genetic abnormalities. A gene on chromosome 21 also appears to be involved in the formation of amyloid, the protein substance found abnormally deposited in the brains of Alzheimer's patients. A number of research findings suggest some genetic relationship between alterations in the gene, the abnormal accumulations of amyloid, and familial Alzheimer's disease (Tanzi, Gusella, et al. 1987; Goldbaber, Lerman, et al. 1987). These relationships have not, however, been established. They may be coincidental. Subsequent research has disputed the possibility that this amyloid gene is duplicated in Alzheimer's disease, a defect that would provide some evidence toward its role as a causative factor.

It is likely that further genetic research will establish more clearly the role that genetic factors play in Alzheimer's disease. Such research also may lead us to new treatments, such as ways to lessen the impact of amyloid on the brain, to frustrate expression of the gene responsible for familial Alzheimer's, or to eliminate other factors required for a genetic predisposition to be awakened. From all evidence, it can take 50 years or more before the genetic defect is manifested as disease. We may also find that other genetic abnormalities make some persons more vulnerable to Alzheimer's. Other types of genetic defects may be involved in causing the disease. An example of such a genetic defect was recently reported by scientists. A blood abnormality found in some cases of Alzheimer's disease may represent an inherited predisposition to the disease or a genetic marker that could predict who might be at risk for the disease (Schmeck, Harold 1987). Persons found to have this blood abnormality tend to develop symptoms of the disease earlier. The rate of the disease's progression is more rapid. This type of finding is valuable for understanding more about the genetic and biological aspects of some cases of Alzheimer's disease. It does not, however, explain most cases.

Relatives of Alzheimer's victims do not have a significantly higher risk of getting the disease.

Once we learn to pinpoint the genetic marker or markers for most cases of inherited Alzheimer's, it also will become possible to identify individuals who are at risk of getting Alzheimer's disease. The idea that Alzheimer's can run in families leads many relatives of Alzheimer's victims to wonder whether they, too, will someday fall prey to the disease. In the great majority of cases, the answer is no. For most close relatives of an Alzheimer's victim, the statistical risk of getting the disease is just very slightly greater than that for the general population. The only persons with real basis for concern are those whose families have documented cases of early-onset Alzheimer's and cases in preceding generations, and who have more than one first-degree relative affected in the current generation.

Unfortunately, it is very difficult to accurately trace family histories of Alzheimer's disease. Since the disease has been generally recognized for only a little more than a decade, it most likely would not have been diagnosed in previous generations. Also, many relatives in previous generations did not live past age 65, when Alzheimer's disease would have been most likely to appear.

Genetic counseling provides more information about risks.

Members of families that do appear to be at risk for Alzheimer's disease may want to consult a genetic counselor. If one's family proves to show an autosomal-dominant pattern of transmission, genetic screening and counseling can provide answers about what might be expected for the future.

The Viral Theory

An extremely slow infectious virus may be the cause. Another theory holds that Alzheimer's disease is caused by an extremely slow, infectious virus that may take several decades to incubate. Other neurological disorders have been found to be caused by such viruses; these include Kuru, Creutzfeldt-Jakob disease, and Gerstmann-Straussler syndrome (Prusiner 1984). These viruses are similar to a viral agent that causes the neurological disorder, scrapie, in sheep and goats. This infectious agent, a prion, is much smaller than conventional viruses.

It has never been shown that Alzheimer's can be transmitted. To prove that such a virus for Alzheimer's disease exists, clinical studies would have to show that the disease can be transmitted. So far, laboratory tests attempting to transmit the disease from brain tissue to animals have failed. It may be, however, that the animals simply were not susceptible to the disease or that the incubation period for the disease is longer than the duration of the studies (Prusiner 1984). (Kuru and Creutzfeldt-Jakob disease, for example, are known to incubate for 20–30 years.) Such a long incubation period would seem consistent with the late age of onset usually found in Alzheimer's.

Some studies have explored the theory that Alzheimer's is caused by a combination of viral and familial/genetic factors. Others have suggested a relationship between amyloid plaques and viral-like agents. Since no hard evidence exists to either confirm or deny the idea that Alzheimer's is caused by a virus, this theory must remain an active area for further research.

The Immune-System Theory

By fighting off bacteria, viruses, and other invaders, the antibodies in the human immune system keep our bodies in good health. Sometimes, however, certain antibodies become confused and react against the body's own cells as though they were invaders. Such misguided antibodies are called "autoimmune antibodies."

Disorder in the immune system is a possible cause. Research has found that the number of autoimmune antibodies in the blood increases with age, and that the elderly tend to get more autoimmune diseases such as cancer, rheumatoid arthritis, and late-onset diabetes (Nandy 1983). Such age-related factors suggest that deterioration of the immune system also may be implicated in Alzheimer's disease. A disorder in the body's immune system, causing the body to attack itself, is another possible cause.

Other indicators point to nonage-related immune system abnormalities. For example, many other neurological diseases—including multiple sclerosis and Huntington's Chorea—are known to involve immune-system alterations, and several studies report findings of marked immune-system irregularities in Alzheimer's patients. As with the theory of viruses, however, more research is needed before immune-system disturbances can be either proved or disproved as a cause of Alzheimer's disease.

The Aluminum Theory

High levels of aluminum in the brain may cause Alzheimer's. Some researchers have theorized that neurofibrillary tangles in Alzheimer's disease and other dementias could be caused by an excess of aluminum in the brain. The concentration of aluminum in the human brain is known to increase with age (Yates 1979; Jenike 1985). Abnormally high levels of aluminum have been found in the brains of persons suffering from other dementias (Thienhaus 1985), though these may well be unrelated to the disease. Together these indications suggest that high levels of aluminum may possibly be related to Alzheimer's disease, though there is certainly no proof of its being a causative factor.

Chelation therapy not proven helpful Some health practitioners advertise chelation therapy and imply that this therapy will reduce aluminum levels and thus improve the impairments that characterize Alzheimer's disease.

There is simply no scientific support for this idea. Often such clinics fail to properly diagnose Alzheimer's disease, assuming that the patient's problems are caused by treatable "vascular dementia." Since chelation therapy is expensive, can produce serious side effects, and has never been proved to help Alzheimer's patients, such treatment should be discouraged. Too often it simply drains the pocketbooks of families desperate for a cure.

Concern about aluminum has led many families to worry about the risks of using aluminum cookware and aluminum-rich antacids and other medications. Though there is no evidence that prolonged use of these products affects Alzheimer's in any way, some researchers suggest that concerned families may wish to request medications with less aluminum from their doctors (Shore and Wyatt 1983) when their medications are extremely high in aluminum.

Psychosocial Factors and Dementia

Negative psychosocial factors create obstacles to caregiving and adjustment.

Psychosocial factors can have powerful effects, both positive and negative, on the lives of people. On the positive side, such things as an adequate income, consistent family support, and a comfortable home environment make caring for a person with dementia much less burdensome. On the negative side, serious health problems, excessive family conflicts, and the absence of daily routines can create obstacles in the care of and adjustment to Alzheimer's disease. Viewed in this context, psychosocial factors can have a definite relationship to how a person with Alzheimer's disease will fare in the long run.

In addition, feelings about the causes of the disease can influence both the caregiver's attitudes and those of the family toward Alzheimer's patients. Family members sometimes wonder whether there is anything in their relative's history that could have caused or contributed to his condition. Family members sometimes blame severe, recent illnesses for precipitating symptoms of dementia. However, if their relative's condition meets criteria for Alzheimer's disease, these other medical problems will have already been ruled out as the cause of the dementia.

Medical trauma can precipitate symptoms. We have seen a few cases in which the aftermath of traumatic medical conditions or reactions to severe losses or psychosocial stressors seem to contribute to the progression of Alzheimer's disease.

Sometimes, a person traumatized by serious medical conditions will begin to exhibit symptoms of dementia. Usually, these symptoms preceded the illness in a very subtle form, but become more pronounced afterwards. Additionally, unlike the hospital-type delirium that occurs with older persons, these symptoms do not disappear. In fact, the person's intellectual and memory abilities not only fail to return but continue to deteriorate. These medical conditions do not cause Alzheimer's disease; they simply precipitate a worsening of the process.

Reactions to the loss of a spouse can hide symptoms of dementia. In the case of reactions to losses or other stressors, the most common situation is the loss of a spouse. Prior to the spouse's death, the surviving spouse will often seem to be handling things relatively well, considering the demands of care and the emotional adjustment. Any subtle symptoms of dementia can be explained as normal reactions to the circumstances. We have also seen cases where the medically ill spouse was the "cognitive" manager of the care situation. He or she kept household activities, bills, and medications under control. These persons, even though physically ill, were caregivers in a sense for the spouse who was later found to have an Alzheimer's-type dementia. When this significant other dies or goes to a nursing home, the spouse left at home may experience substantial loss of organization, routine, and support. Grief and/or depression may be observed.

The grief or depression may not immediately appear, but it may emerge later as reactions to coping with dramatic life changes. It may be difficult initially to determine whether the impairments of memory and intellectual abilities are the symptoms of dementia or reactions to what has happened. Pseudodementia may be present in the form of depression, which can coexist with Alzheimer's disease.

Medical problems and significant psychosocial losses can enhance the symptoms of Alzheimer's disease. Again, these events do not cause the disease; they accentuate symptoms that were already developing insidiously.

No connection between past events and Alzheimer's disease

Families sometimes try to blame psychosocial stressors or other past events in a person's life for Alzheimer's disease, even though there is no connection. Relatives' beliefs at times center on things that should or should not have been done (e.g., he should have worked harder, or he worked too hard). Family members may point to some specific event in the past that brought about changes in their relative's behavior. For example, they may say their relative never was the same after his parents died or after he lost a job 15 years ago or after he had a knock-down-drag-out fight with his brother. They may try to resurrect these problems as explanations for Alzheimer's disease. Behavioral changes, indeed, may have occurred in their relative after these kinds of events, yet there is no reason to believe these events caused the degenerative brain disease.

When a person affected by Alzheimer's disease has had a troubled life long before the illness began, there may be considerable hard feelings and conflicts within his family. Family members may be both bitter and resentful of things they believe their affected relative did to them or others. In this case, what the family says is the cause for Alzheimer's disease, they really think of as deserved punishment. Hostility and anger can erupt, and caregiving may be difficult for such family members to provide. This is a family situation that is at risk for abuse to occur. However, the affected relative's "sin" of commission or omission did not cause the Alzheimer's-type condition.

The family adjustment process can sometimes bring up beliefs about why the loved one has developed Alzheimer's disease. These beliefs, unlike those just described, usually represent family members' attempts to come to terms with this illness.

A history of psychiatric problems does not increase risk.

People who have had psychiatric problems throughout their lives are not necessarily more susceptible to Alzheimer's disease. However, some families may believe that psychiatric illnesses, such as chronic depression, are responsible for later brain disorders. There is virtually no evidence for this contention. One research report suggests that persons with Alzheimer's disease do seem to have a higher incidence of psychiatric episodes, especially depression, which occur much earlier than the onset of the disease's symptoms (Agbayewa 1986).

Psychiatric episodes often are precursors to more obvious symptoms of dementia. The author of this research suggests that the psychiatric episodes could conceivably represent prodromal stages of the illness. In addition to depression, paranoid disorders were strongly implicated as potential forerunners of the Alzheimer's-type dementia (Agbayewa 1986). This area of research should be continued; however, the reported findings should be viewed cautiously.

Psychiatric symptoms can be manifested during the course of Alzheimer's disease. Delusions, hallucinations, agitation, anxiety, depression, and catastrophic reactions can all occur. Psychiatric manifestations, their intensity and duration can vary from one individual to another. The environment, which includes the family, has some influence.

Sensory impairments contribute to hallucinations and delusions. Sensory impairments such as existing visual and hearing problems contribute to individual variations. For instance, persons with significant hearing impairment can be more susceptible to auditory hallucinations, even when they do not have Alzheimer's disease. Limitations in reasoning and interpretation of sounds in Alzheimer's create a greater chance of hallucinations, and delusions sometimes develop out of these hallucinations.

Personality factors enter into psychiatric symptoms which accompany Alzheimer's disease. By the time an individual develops this condition, his personality traits are well defined. Enduring characteristics of the person, how he behaves socially, and how he typically responds to situations are indicators of his personality. Suspicious and paranoid types may become more agitated and distrustful when they have Alzheimer's disease. A person who has always been dependent will become more dependent and insecure.

Familiar, well-organized, comfortable environment minimizes coping problems.

Environmental factors, including physical arrangement and social and psychological overtones, exert considerable influences on how individuals cope with Alzheimer's disease. The caregiving environment will also determine to a degree the effectiveness and endurance of the caregiver. A familiar, well-organized, and comfortable environment can be supportive of Alzheimer's care. Good lighting during the day and enough lighting at night to help the patient find the bathroom can be helpful. Later, signs can be used to indicate the bathroom door. A poster with important reminders, names, and phone numbers can increase the security of some Alzheimer's patients when the caregiver must be gone for a short while. The house can be secured at night to prevent the patient's wandering outside the home. Additionally, the household can be run in a calm, relaxed manner to reduce unnecessary noise and unsettling distractions.

Social contact is important for both patient and caregiver.

Complete social isolation is harmful for both the caregiver and the patient. Outside social contact need not be lengthy for the Alzheimer's patient, but some degree of consistency from friends and other family helps maintain a sense of a social bond. For example, the length of visits can be preset and arranged to include both the patient and the caregiver. When the patient begins to tire and withdraw somewhat from the conversation, the visitor can spend some focused time with the caregiver, satisfying both persons' need for social interaction. At times, those who have Alzheimer's disease are self-conscious about their limitations and may leave the room even when visitors are still there. Both visitors and caregiver should accept the departure without protest; the patient should not be forced to stay. Additionally, caregivers need to reassure the affected relatives that they are loved and accepted in spite of the disease.

Psychological environment

The psychological environment should be encouraging and supportive. A calm atmosphere has a more relaxing effect on both the patient and the caregiver. Of course, some stimulation and activity must be preserved according to the capabilities of the person receiving the care. Too many demands may create more restlessness and agitation. The affected relative should no longer be held accountable for many of his mistakes and errors in judgment. The caregiver's insistent correction can result in more reactive responses from the patient. Any opportunity to support the shrinking self-esteem of the Alzheimer's patient must be acted upon. Meaningful rewards are important, even for helping with the smallest of tasks.

In this book, a great deal of emphasis is placed on the beliefs of family members concerning the changed behavior of their affected relative. When families can understand more of their relative's behavior from the perspective of brain impairment, they can relate more successfully to that behavior. Their responses can be more sensitive without as much anger and frustration. Uninformed and overburdened caregivers have attributed intricate intellectual plans to loved ones, believing that the brain-impaired person consciously followed these plans to get what he wanted or to repay the caregiver for some supposed insult. It is questionable whether an Alzheimer's patient can respond in such a premeditated manner. It is more likely he is reacting to something in the environment or to his own misinterpretations.

Isolation has a profound effect on elderly persons living alone. From our community work in geriatric mental health, we have seen the profound effects isolation can have on some elderly who live alone. They are referred to us for treatment when they seem to be a danger to themselves or seem unable to provide for their most basic needs. Most often family or neighbors notice unusual or frightening behavior and call us for help. When we go to the home to check out these reports, we often find the house in disarray, cans of open food on the cabinets, decomposing items in the refrigerator, and unopened take-out lunches from the senior center on the counter. Sometimes we find the person just lying on the floor in a heap. In some instances, these people may be defensive when they see us, but often they try to be cordial and friendly. They are bewildered by troubles they cannot seem to handle on their own, but they are frightened to allow strangers to help them (a reasonable response even if the strangers are part of a geriatric mental health team).

In these kinds of cases, symptoms of dementia are often present. Many of these persons will eventually be diagnosed as having Alzheimer's disease. Occasionally, reversible medical conditions or pseudodementia are found to be responsible for the functional impairments.

Hearing and visual impairments contribute to isolation.
Hearing and visual impairments often contribute to isolation in the elderly. Sensory and social deprivation are known to have significant impact on a person's functioning, and in the elderly individual with dementia, they suggest that psychosocial factors play a role in precipitating delusions and hallucinations. Interestingly, the hallucinations and delusions in this context may be attempts at creating stimulation in a world that has shrunk to the parameters of a couple of rooms. The isolated person with dementia is stuck between the insecurity of memory problems and the fear of other people taking over his life.

Reaction to nursing home placement is influenced by benefits perceived in the move.
Eventually the Alzheimer's patient may have to be placed in a nursing home or other 24-hour facility. Placing a family member in a nursing home is a difficult decision for families involved in Alzheimer's care. However, relocation effects on the patient are influenced by the person's perception of loss of control along with other aspects of the move.

Thus it is how the living situation changes, not the change itself that is important. If the relocation improves the person's living situation, its effects will not be detrimental. For example, persons make a better adjustment to a nursing home relocation if they perceive the care as better, have easier accessibility to their physician, have meaningful things to do, and have the opportunity to make friends.

The factors above increase security and, consequently, the person's sense of control because there is more positively defined predictability in his life. However, of the factors that indicate quality, one is more significant than all the others: the extent of social support the person perceives himself to receive. It is the emotional response induced by the change, not the change itself, that is vital (Henry 1986).

More advanced Alzheimer's patients do not have the intellectual capacity necessary to adjust to a new environment without considerable assistance. However, they may relate most often—at a basic emotional level—to what is happening to and around them, as their ability to reason and make intellectual judgments fades.

These observations have applications to caregiving even when there is no relocation in the immediate future. A strong sense of social support is critical to persons with Alzheimer's disease whether they are living in nursing homes or in their own homes. Deprived environments can precipitate "excessive disability" and "learned helplessness," while supportive and stimulating environments encourage individuals to maintain more control of their lives and be a little more involved in the world outside of themselves.

Uncertainty about the causes of Alzheimer's disease has negative effects.

Not knowing what causes Alzheimer's is a psychosocial factor of the disease which often has negative effects on dementia patients and their caregivers. For the most part, we do not know what puts a person at risk for Alzheimer's disease. One exception is some genetic risks of inheritance in a small group of families in which the affected relative develops the disease before age 70 and another relative is also affected. Some research suggests that persons who have had previous head injuries may have a slightly greater risk for developing Alzheimer's disease.

There is not sufficient evidence to state that Alzheimer's affects one race of people more than another. It occurs fairly uniformly. Although more women than men have been reported to develop Alzheimer's in the past, this observation seems to be modified as more men live longer. The difference is probably marginal. Some persons believe nutrition and diet might play a role in the disease, but this has not been substantiated by research. Poor nutrition can result in conditions that produce symptoms of dementia in the elderly, for example, pernicious anemia. However, there is no evidence that nutritional deficiencies cause Alzheimer's disease.

Many of the abnormalities found in the Alzheimer's brain are associated with aging, and the incidence of Alzheimer's disease increases with age. However, these facts do not indicate that aging itself causes Alzheimer's disease. There may be age-related mechanisms which contribute to Alzheimer's appearance, or perhaps there are several mechanisms that interact to cause the disease. When we know what these factors are, it may be possible to develop preventive approaches based on risk factors.

Community resources need to be increased. For this long moment in time, while we wait for a cure or treatment, we must use what we know to make the lives of individuals with Alzheimer's disease as well as the family caregivers safer and more meaningful. Other approaches to long-term care must be developed. Many communities are still lacking the resources to support Alzheimer's services, such as day and respite care. Families often feel less helpless in dealing with this illness if they are involved in support groups. Political action has already paid off for Alzheimer's research, but more research and care options are needed. Families can work with their own legislators or city officials to gather more support for funding vital services. Area Agencies on Aging can help develop options.

Families must not be afraid to seek available help. Just doing something about the situation often counteracts feelings of helplessness and hopelessness. Families must be willing to seek help when they need it, particularly when help is available. Certainly Alzheimer's disease can be described in tragic terms, but there are other tragedies which can often be prevented. One example is the suffering that families experience when they are unwilling to seek help that is available. Another example is the suffering added to the lives of persons experiencing or dealing with Alzheimer's disease by insensitive professionals who project their own hopelessness into the lives of those they are charged with helping. Such needless pain can and must be prevented.

5

SIX COMMON MYTHS ABOUT ALZHEIMER'S

Families hold misconceptions. Many misconceptions exist about the nature of Alzheimer's disease. Lacking adequate information about the disease, families commonly hold mistaken notions about the disease itself, old age, and their own role in caring for the person with Alzheimer's. In addition, they may harbor unnecessary fears about the likelihood that they will inherit the disease from their relative.

Because our beliefs are the basis for our actions, it is important that families have an accurate understanding of Alzheimer's and its significance. The following are some of the most common myths about Alzheimer's, followed by a correct assessment of the pertinent issues.

Myth 1: Alzheimer's Symptoms Are a Normal Sign of Old Age

Alzheimer's should not be confused with the aging process. Some of the early symptoms of Alzheimer's, such as forgetfulness, do correspond to our common notions of aging; but Alzheimer's is a disease and should not be confused with the aging process. This becomes clear as the disease progresses, and the victim's deterioration becomes more dramatic.

Old-age forgetfulness is benign. In terms of memory loss, for example, it is true that a degree of increased forgetfulness commonly accompanies aging. Older persons may find it more difficult to recall the details of past events. However, the memory loss caused by Alzheimer's is far more severe and progressive in nature. Eventually the disease destroys not just the memory of details but all memory of the event itself. The person in time will forget not only the events of the past but what she did that morning, who her spouse is, where she lives, even her own name. These are not the normal consequences of aging.

Myth 2:   Senility Is the Usual Cause of Problems in Old Age

Senility obscures real illnesses and problems of aging.
Senility is a blanket term that has long been used to cover a wide-ranging variety of symptoms. In this sense it is a damaging notion and a term to be avoided. An assumed diagnosis of senility obscures the real problem at hand and increases the difficulty of getting correct treatment for the older person's condition or impairment. The older person may suffer along assuming her condition is irreversible, when treatment may in fact be readily available. In addition, the myth of senility reinforces the negative and mistaken belief that all persons must become helpless and useless with age.

Common hearing and visual problems produce misleading views of older persons.
If an older person has difficulty relating to others or conducting her affairs, many problems other than senility or Alzheimer's disease may be the source. For example, the person may suffer from impaired hearing or vision. Her failure to clearly follow a conversation or respond to something in the environment may make it seem that her thought processes are impaired, when actually she has simply not seen or heard what happened. Additionally, the impaired person may begin to avoid situations where her problem is most apparent or troublesome. A person who is hard of hearing may avoid crowds, while a person with poor sight may become confused in social situations because everyone's face looks the same. Often older persons are unwilling to admit these impairments, which can add to confusion about the source of their problems.

Medical problems produce emotional and behavioral changes labeled as senility.

Medical conditions also may be at the root of the older person's problems. Congestive heart failure may cause weakness, fatigue, mental confusion, forgetfulness, and other symptoms mistaken for senility. Hyperthyroidism may cause apathy, depression, lethargy, impaired memory, and slow responses in the elderly. Hypothyroidism has similar symptoms in the elderly, with weakness and fatigue a little more prominent. Both of these illnesses have a slow, progressive onset similar to that of Alzheimer's disease. Persons suffering from these problems should receive a full medical evaluation, and family members should not just assume that the problem is old age.

Other conditions that may be confused with Alzheimer's include B-12 deficiencies, pernicious anemia, electrolyte imbalances, normal pressure hydrocephalus, hypoglycemia, and a range of infections. Infections of the urinary system, for example, may cause confusion, apathy, and inattentiveness before other symptoms are apparent. It is therefore essential that experienced medical personnel rule out all other possible causes for the older person's problems before arriving at a diagnosis of Alzheimer's.

Medications create Alzheimer's-type symptoms.

Often medication prescribed for a medical condition can cause side effects similar to Alzheimer's symptoms, such as confusion, forgetfulness, tremors, and slower responses. This can be a particular problem when the older person is taking several medications at one time to treat different conditions. If problems are apparent, they should be brought promptly to the attention of the doctor or doctors involved. When a number of doctors and pharmacies are involved with different medications, there is a greater chance that medication-related problems will develop. It is therefore extremely important to provide all professionals involved with an up-to-date regimen of medications.

Depression is often mistaken for senility.

Psychological problems such as depression often are passed off as senility as well. It is common for older persons to experience some depression as they face the loss of health, friends, spouse, home, as well as their own death. Such major life changes late in life may lead to mental conditions requiring a psychiatrist's care, such as severe depression, anxiety, or paranoia. The person may not seem "crazy," but fear and insecurity in the face of real losses or perceived threats may be interfering with her ability to effectively cope with life.

Depression accentuates other difficulties.
Depression can in turn lead to complaints about memory problems. The person may see even minor memory lapses as evidence that she is becoming senile. In fact, however, she may simply be suffering from lapses in attention and concentration caused by the depression. One difference between the symptoms of depression and those of Alzheimer's is that, while the depressed person may not recognize her depression, she will rarely deny the resulting problems. Alzheimer's victims, on the other hand, tend to deny all evidence of the disease.

A belief in senility stops people from seeking help.
The myth of senility and the lack of dignity associated with it often prevent older persons from seeking treatment for conditions that are in fact reversible. Family members should encourage older persons to seek medical treatment for the problems they encounter and should not let them assume that senility is a necessary consequence of old age.

Myth 3: Nothing Can Be Done for the Alzheimer's Victim

Proper care is important in the management of the illness.
It is true that at present we have no cure for Alzheimer's disease. The disease is progressive and leads ultimately to death. However, there is much that can be done to make the victim's last months or years more meaningful, pleasant, and comfortable.

Medical care
Alzheimer's patients benefit from both proper medical care and informed behavior management. Thus the family should involve health

professionals in their victim's care as early as possible, and they should continue to seek professional opinions throughout the disease.

Psychiatric care

Psychiatrists and other mental health professionals can successfully treat the depression or other psychological symptoms that frequently develop. Doctors and nutritionists can provide help with meal preparation, special diets, and nutritional supplements as the person's appetite and eating abilities deteriorate. Careful attention to the use of medications will prevent unnecessary and prolonged side effects.

Other medical problems coexist.

Treatment of coexisting medical problems is also very important. It should not be assumed that all of the person's physical and mental symptoms are caused by the disease. Persons with Alzheimer's are especially vulnerable to the common viruses, colds, and infections that affect us all, including pneumonia, and these conditions should receive prompt medical attention.

Myth 4: Alzheimer's Is Strictly a Mental Illness

Psychiatric symptoms

Many of the changes initially observed in the Alzheimer's patient seem to be personality disorders or other psychological problems. Furthermore, because Alzheimer's disease primarily affects the brain, it is in a sense a "mental" illness. However, Alzheimer's disease is a degenerative medical condition and not a psychiatric disorder.

Psychiatric symptoms are a significant part of the illness. As the brain gradually loses its capacity to perform normal functions we take for granted, the individual becomes increasingly insecure and unable to relate to her daily world. In time her personality is completely altered, and she truly becomes a "different person" than the loved one we have always known.

Insurance views the illness as psychiatric. Because society's recognition of the medical nature of the disease is fairly recent, however, Alzheimer's may be regarded at times as a psychiatric condition. Persons financially dependent on insurance or Medicaid programs, for example, may find that they do not meet the "medical" requirements that make them eligible for long-term care. It is to be hoped that these requirements and attitudes will change as the understanding of Alzheimer's becomes more widespread.

Diagnostic findings of good health are misleading. The impression that Alzheimer's is a mental illness may be supported when a diagnosis of general "good health" is coupled with a diagnosis of Alzheimer's disease. What medical professionals mean by such a diagnosis, however, is that no other medical problems have been found, or other conditions are so successfully controlled that the individual is in otherwise satisfactory health.

Myth 5: Only the Family Should Care for the Alzheimer's Victim

Family care is supportive and necessary. In most cases, it is certainly best if the affected person can stay at home with her spouse or family as long as possible. The love and regular interaction a family can provide usually helps the person retain her abilities longer and helps ease her difficult adjustment to the disease.

Other resources make a big difference. However, not all spouses or children have the resources to care properly for their loved one. Even those who do have the resources eventually may have to call upon outside care when the disease reaches its later stages and caregiving becomes an utterly exhausting experience.

Caregivers should be careful about overinvolvement. Overinvolvement, or the feeling that the caregiver must do everything herself, is a common reaction to the disease. Often it represents a stage in the family member's adjustment to the disease (see Chapter 7). The caregiver imagines that she can hold back the disease by doing everything herself, and her grief leads her to become extremely protective of the victim. She may also feel reluctant to seek outside help because of shame and the stigmas associated with mental conditions.

Primary caregivers must accept help. However, the family, and in particular the primary caregiver, must learn to accept help. The burden of caring for an Alzheimer's patient can otherwise cause serious problems for the caregiver and alienate her from friends and family who want to share the caregiving role. The caregiver should not hesitate to call upon community resources as well, such as those discussed in detail in Chapter 10. Without these resources, the burden of care can become overwhelming.

Myth 6:   All Relatives of Alzheimer's Victims Are Likely to Inherit the Disease

Risk of contracting the disease is not high for most families of victims. It is common for relatives of Alzheimer's victims to worry that they may have a genetic predisposition toward the disease. However, current research indicates that the risk for children, parents, and siblings of Alzheimer's victims is no higher or only slightly higher than the risk for the general population. More research into genetic and other factors relevant to Alzheimer's disease must be conducted, however, before risk factors can be positively identified.

Alzheimer's does not follow any hard and fast rules. Alzheimer's does not follow any hard and fast rules. It hits people at different ages, progresses at different rates, and affects each individual somewhat differently, which makes generalizations difficult. In addition, the difficulty in diagnosing the disease means that other medical conditions (e.g., Pick's disease, Creutzfeldt-Jakob disease) may have affected relatives thought to have had Alzheimer's.

**Minimal in-
creased risk
for family
members**
Some factors do suggest a higher family risk, but they must be interpreted in view of the history of the individual's illness, age at onset, and the known diagnosis of similar conditions in any other relatives. Of course, it can be difficult to determine whether relatives had Alzheimer's, because conditions that may have had similarities to Alzheimer's were diagnosed as everything from senility to hardening of the arteries.

The risk for family members with a relative who has Alzheimer's depends on several factors. If the onset of the illness occurs at a younger age, relatives are at a slightly higher risk. If more than one person in a family is afflicted with the disease, others in the family also have a higher degree of risk. In both cases, the disease has often been observed to be more severe.

Dr. Leonard L. Heston gives examples of three types of family risk situations based on severity (Heston 1985). Risk for children of Alzheimer's victims is not known, but it is probably about the same as that for siblings and parents.

Type I

- Onset of illness occurs at age 70 +
- No other relative is affected
- Risk begins at age 65 for siblings, parents
- Risk at age 80 would be 12 percent in siblings/parents of affected person.

Type II

- Onset of illness occurs at less than age 70
- No other relative is affected
- Risk begins at age 60 for siblings/parents
- Risk by age 80 would be 16 percent for siblings/parents.

Type III

- Onset of illness occurs at less than age 70
- Another relative is affected by the disease
- Risk begins at age 45 for siblings/parents
- Risk begins at age 65 for uncles, aunts, nephews, nieces, grandchildren, of affected relatives
- Risk by age 55 is 8 percent, by age 65 is 16 percent, by age 80 is 28 percent, and by age 95 is 40 percent for siblings/parents
- More distant relatives in this type of family have a slightly higher risk than that of the general population.

Family risk generally is no higher than that for the general population.

For most families of Alzheimer's victims, the genetic risk for contracting the disease is not much higher than the risk for the general population. Only members of a Type III family have cause for serious concern about genetic predisposition to the illness. Genetic research findings might best be viewed as tentative, and members of a family with an Alzheimer's victim should not be overly concerned about contracting the disease.

6

COPING: A STEP-BY-STEP GUIDE TO THE CAREGIVER'S EXPERIENCE

A hypothetical case history — Eleanor is becoming increasingly concerned about her husband Bill. He has made some errors in his checkbook, which are uncharacteristic, and twice recently he has gotten lost driving in unfamiliar parts of town. Yet when she brings her concerns up, he becomes angry and denies everything. At first, she associated these problems with getting old. Bill does have early cataracts and does not see well. But now he is becoming suspicious of her and the neighbors. Recently she was shocked when he confronted a neighbor about stealing tools out of the garage. He had never done anything like that before.

During the last few years, Eleanor has heard a great deal about Alzheimer's disease. She is afraid that something like that might be happening to Bill. Her husband is slowly changing, and she feels a growing pressure to do something. But what? Should she talk to the family doctor or a psychiatrist? It has always been difficult to get Bill to see a doctor, and Bill keeps insisting that he has no problems. Bill's behavior is becoming embarrassing to Eleanor, which makes her reluctant to do things with her friends. She does not know how to tell the children about her fears, and since they both live out of state, they have not seen for themselves what is happening to their father. Whenever Eleanor thinks about the changes in Bill, she feels alone and afraid.

Responding to Alzheimer's symptoms is difficult. — Eleanor's predicament is typical of the difficult situation in which relatives of persons in the early stages of Alzheimer's often find themselves. They feel certain that something is very wrong, but they do not know what they should do to help. Never having experienced anything like this before and afraid that the problem may be more serious than they can bear, they feel at a loss to identify the first step.

Knowing what lies ahead helps. This chapter seeks to alleviate the confusion and anxiety that caregivers experience by offering a step-by-step guide to the process of coping with Alzheimer's disease. It outlines the steps that caregivers will need to take and offers helpful, practical advice for what to do at each stage. By clearly identifying the disease process and the challenges that lie ahead for the caregiver, the information in this chapter aims to relieve the anxiety caregivers feel in facing an unknown threat. The following are the steps discussed in depth in this chapter.

1. Noticing initial symptoms
2. Confirming suspicions
3. Seeking information
4. Taking action
5. Weighing findings
6. Identifying resources
7. Planning care
8. Managing caregiver stress

1. Noticing Initial Symptoms

All illnesses have symptoms. If the problem is a physical one, the symptoms are likely to be familiar physical complaints such as fever, headache, nausea, fatigue, and specific areas of pain. The signs of mental illness can be more difficult to identify, yet symptoms are still present. Persons suffering from depression, for example, may not recognize that they are depressed, yet they often report symptoms. Similarly, persons with Alzheimer's may experience symptoms but fail to attribute them to a brain condition.

**Early symp-
toms may not
clearly suggest
Alzheimer's
disease.**

With Alzheimer's, symptoms observed early in the illness are likely to be behavioral or emotional, and the person's distress is usually psychological. He probably will not associate his initial problems with an intellectual function such as memory or suspect that a serious illness is the cause. Though a spouse or other relative may observe slight changes in the person's normal behavior, it is difficult to take these changes seriously at first.

**Denial of
symptoms is
common.**

The affected person may feel that acknowledging his difficulties would create unnecessary worries for his family or place his job in jeopardy. He may feel that he can overcome these problems if he tries harder.

Often, when he discovers that he can do little about his memory problems, he will become noticeably anxious, frustrated, and irritable with the possibility of depression developing. It is common for the affected person to point out memory lapses of other family members to distract attention from his own growing difficulties.

**Symptoms be-
come harder
to ignore.**

However, the person's memory problems, as well as his emotional and behavioral reactions, will begin eventually to create genuine concern among family members. They will begin to wonder if perhaps the changes and deficiencies they are noticing might be symptoms of something larger.

2. Confirming Suspicions

**Families must
seek profes-
sional help.**

Families usually discuss early concerns with other family and friends first. As initial doubts become more persistent, they generally feel a need to share their concerns with a health professional who can positively confirm or deny their suspicions.

It is important to consult a health professional as soon as possible, for a preliminary medical consultation will

- Clarify the seriousness of the problems
- Verify the need for action
- Ensure prompt treatment if the condition is not in fact Alzheimer's.

A professional provides both medical information and emotional support.   Often, it is difficult to get the person to agree to see a doctor, and many families are reluctant to take a relative to a health professional without consent. When this problem arises, the family may wish to consult a doctor or a mental health professional on their own. Contact with a professional can

- Give initial feedback on whether the symptoms described sound like those associated with Alzheimer's
- Suggest where to go for a comprehensive evaluation of the relative's condition, and explain the costs and time involved
- Address the fears, doubts, and confusion of family members about what needs to be done. (This area alone justifies contact with a professional familiar with Alzheimer's disease.)

If the family can provide the professional with a list of problems and examples of symptoms observed, this will help the professional make a determination of a person's condition.

Use of Behavior Profile   Included in the appendix is a "Behavior Profile" which is a comprehensive listing of difficulties ranging from orientation to behavior problems. This scale is helpful for families in documenting problems and their frequency. The profile also provides the caregiver with an opportunity to determine how stressful he finds a particular behavior. It will be useful later in the illness to determine the amount of assistance a person requires and specific behaviors that require more intervention and supportive counseling to relieve the stress surrounding such behaviors.

Families should establish a clear history of symptoms.

The history of symptoms and problems is extremely important in making an accurate diagnosis. Families should note how long they have observed various symptoms in their relative. A number of illnesses such as depression and strokes without motor impairment have symptoms that are very similar to those characteristic of Alzheimer's disease. A good history of such symptoms will reflect whether they developed suddenly or over an extended period. Such information becomes significant in the evaluation of this illness.

3. Seeking Information

Community resources provide information and support.

In addition to consulting a family doctor, neurologist, psychiatrist, or other mental health professional, the family may wish to seek information on Alzheimer's disease from an Alzheimer's Family Support Group or an Alzheimer's Resource Center. Family support meetings can put a family in touch with vital local resources as well as with professionals who are experienced in diagnosing Alzheimer's disease.

4. Taking Action

A full evaluation involves several health professionals.

An appointment with the family physician may be the starting point for the evaluative process, with basic tests ordered. Often the physician may refer his patient to another professional, such as a neurologist, psychiatrist, or a mental health center for evaluation.

Since the family has decided to act, they want results and some answers. What will help? What can be done to manage the situation even though no cure exists? The family probably expects a medication to manage symptoms. The family's need for information accelerates after the implications of the diagnosis are recognized.

Seeking a second opinion may be necessary. If a physician gives the diagnosis of Alzheimer's after minimal testing, the family may experience a letdown that can create distrust, lack of confidence in the physician, and real dissatisfaction. A similar situation exists when incorrect diagnosis of senility or hardening of the arteries is given to informed family members who are keenly aware of their loved one's extreme degree of impairment. Not all doctors are experts in diagnosing and managing the disease, and families should not hesitate to seek a second opinion if they feel dissatisfied with the first diagnosis. If Alzheimer's is suspected, a doctor with a particular expertise in the disease should be consulted—even if this means traveling to another city.

5. Weighing Findings

Families must evaluate the implications of a diagnosis. After initial diagnostic evaluations have been completed, family members are faced with several tasks including:

a. Questioning the diagnosis and considering the need for a second opinion

b. Understanding the implications of this diagnosis, particularly when confusing, conflicting, or inaccurate information and advice from both professional and nonprofessional sources must be reconciled

c. Reaching a family consensus about what needs to be done now, and in the future, and by whom

d. Deciding whether others should be told about the Alzheimer's condition.

6. Identifying Resources

Alzheimer's as yet cannot be cured. However, some of the related problems can be managed and even treated with medication and proper behavioral management.

Families must realistically assess resources. Before embarking upon a plan of management for the disease and care for the person affected, family members need to realistically assess their personal resources in both emotional and financial terms and examine those offered in the community. Personal resources in this sense are determined by the following factors:

a. The physical health of the most likely primary caregiver

b. The availability of community support and resources

c. The caregiver's living situation and the proximity of other involved family members

d. The family's financial resources and the victim's eligibility for publicly funded services

e. The strength of the caregiver's marital relationship (Can it withstand the stresses of continuous caregiving?)

f. The availability of transportation

g. The availability of family, friends, or paid help to take over care of patient for several hours at least twice a week

h. The availability of persons who fill the role of confidant.

Compensating for changes in one's personal/social supports   Caregivers must realize the support system of friends and family that has helped them in previous times of trouble may not be enough to get them through the stresses of caring for their loved one. Alzheimer's caregiving can last a long time. The family caregiver must assess the potential support available during the caregiving process as realistically as possible and begin to find replacements for the emotional support previously provided by the victim himself.

The caregiver can use the "Personal/Social Support Resources" form in the appendix to assess the degree of support that is currently available. Caregivers must realize that they need support for themselves, too. If the affected family member has been the primary source of support, new resources must be actively sought out.

7. Planning Care

A plan is necessary.   Planning the care of an Alzheimer's victim can seem to be a confusing and perhaps even unnecessary task (especially when the patient is not exhibiting serious management problems). However, as time moves on and the disease progresses, it will become obvious that a plan is necessary.

A home-care planning list is in the Appendix.   To begin the care-planning process, a "Family In-Home Behavior Care List" is included in the appendix. The questions on the list will help a family identify areas in which their relative needs assistance and how much assistance is needed. Caregivers must begin to prioritize needs, and they must decide who best can deliver the needed help. They must realize that their lives are changed by the disease, and they must change their approaches accordingly.

Problem behavior needs careful consideration.

Other approaches to problem-solving should be considered in family care planning.

a. When do problem behaviors occur, and what else is happening when these problems surface? (For example, is the person more difficult and irritable when the television is playing loudly?)

b. What occurs before or after the undesired behavior? Are these events or conditions producing and rewarding the undesired behavior?

c. How frequently does the problem occur? Is it really that big a problem?

d. How severe or dangerous is the problem?

e. Can advance planning reduce opportunities for the problem behavior to occur?

Case example of problem-solving

Emma started calling for her husband at night after she had gone to bed. He usually helped her to bed about 10 P.M. and then stayed up a while alone. She usually fell asleep before she awoke in a panic calling for her husband, somewhat confused. Her husband always turned the light off before going into the den for his quiet time. Because she was so afraid, her husband always ran to her rescue, most often holding her and falling asleep with her. Night after night, she became frightened when she awoke in the dark. As a consequence, her husband had very little time to himself.

Emma's husband realized he was reinforcing her behavior—the calls at night increased. He also realized that waking in the dark might be frightening to Emma. To deal with the problem he did several things.

■ He spent more intimate time with his wife before she went to sleep

■ He left a lamp on in the bedroom while she was asleep

- When she called for him, he called back to her, reassuring her he was just down the hall in the den. Most of the time Emma went back to sleep, and her husband could continue relaxing alone.

8. Managing Caregiver Stress

Stress from caregiving is not necessarily a result of the Alzheimer's condition. Too often the stress of caregiving is attributed solely to the condition of the relative with Alzheimer's. As his condition worsens, the stress experienced by the family caregiver increases. This point of view fails to appreciate other aspects of the caregiving situation, which in turn can make it more difficult for the caregiver to cope effectively with the needs of his relative. More contact from friends and relatives provides for the social and emotional support needs that have increased during the caregiver's physical isolation of more solitary care situations. Utilization of available resources is another factor influencing the caregivers perception of stress. Resources can actually allow the caregiver to participate more in the community.

Other factors influence caregiver stress. The age of the caregiver may influence the degree of stress he experiences. Younger caregivers may have other career and family responsibilities that conflict with full assumption of the caregiving role. The type of role change created by caregiving also influences the degree of stress that will be experienced. For example, female caregivers may resent a return to the caregiver role itself when it had been abandoned for a career after children were grown. Some men, on the other hand, may view the role change associated with a new "provider" role more satisfying. Nurturing his ill spouse offers the male a way to repay his wife for her earlier role in family nurturing.

Caregivers need to help themselves. The stresses of caregiving are not simply the result of the continued deterioration of the relative affected. The well-being of the family caregiver is essential. One of the purposes for an Alzheimer's Family Support Group is to help family members cope successfully with the illness. Counseling also can be sought. Caregivers may prevent some stress by utilizing their personal/social support resources.

Caregivers can do much to help themselves. They should explore community services, and they must recognize their limitations, especially during a long period of intense care. Without outside support, caregivers can develop stress-induced illnesses such as depression and anxiety (see Chapter 3 on Depression and Alzheimer's). Medical problems such as hypertension, diabetes, and heart conditions may worsen because of prolonged stress and poorer self-care.

A stress test is included in the appendix. The "Care Management Stress" scale included in the appendix can help families identify specific stress areas. The areas include stress created by family expectations, isolation, problem behaviors, an uncertain future, and the inherent burden of day-to-day care. In responding to the questions, the caregiver should note the frequency of each response and his emotional response to each statement and make care decisions accordingly.

A stress scale for institutional caregivers is a good preventive tool. Staff of nursing homes and other institutionals also can experience stress as they see the consequences of the illness daily. A "Staff Stress Measure" is included in the appendix. Training and other educational opportunities can help staff understand Alzheimer's, deal with behavior effectively and compassionately, and manage the stress associated with such care.

Both the "Care Management Stress" scale and the "Staff Stress Measure" can be scored. The higher the score, the higher is the potential for stress. More importantly, caregivers can identify particularly stressful areas and give them more attention.

Managing stress is an ongoing activity.

Managing stress is an ongoing activity. Different features of the patient's progressive condition precipitate new problems and stressors. For example, the first time the Alzheimer's patient fails to recognize his spouse may be so shocking that the caregiver's adjustment is set back considerably.

Stress is likely to grow.

As the patient's condition worsens, the stress felt by the caregiver is likely to grow. He should therefore be willing to continuously reassess the possibility of seeking outside help in some form. These resources range from day or respite care to psychiatric hospitalization or nursing home admission. Outpatient mental health services also should be considered as the burdens placed on the caregiver mount.

Look for positive experiences in caregiving.

There are many ways to change the negatives of this illness into some unexpected positives. Opportunities actually surface from the most unexpected situations, which may lead to new experiences or back to old experiences and activities that seemed to have been lost.

Some examples of the positive aspects of caregiving

Thomas became the caregiver for his wife about six months ago. He had been doing the cooking and washing. Then his wife required help with bathing and dressing as well. His "hands-on" care began to increase.

A chance to return years of loving care

After years of working hard while his wife Janet reared their six children (and some would say their seven grandchildren), Thomas saw that he had the chance to give back to Janet all the love and care she had so willing given to her entire family.

A chance to gain unexpected support   Johnnie was almost devastated when she first learned that her husband Ted had Alzheimer's disease. Months later, she became involved in a local Alzheimer's Family Support Group. Over the next few months, she came to know a number of other people in situations like hers. They became close friends and confidantes—something she never thought she would have. For two years she benefitted from their support and concern, and they from hers. When Ted died, these friends stood by her along with her family.

FEELINGS

I've had my wounds
and I'm not sure
anyone knows how to heal them.

The doctors and my friends,
family and others
tell me—

"You've lost so much,
you've nursed your loved one
through a baffling disease—

"You've been ignored
drawn taut—
suffered and cried.

"Now that he
is in a nursing home
and you have help
in caring for him,
you are now free
to live your own life.

"Get out and go—
join clubs—be with people—
develop some hobbies—
travel a bit."

I'm trying—I'm trying—
I know they love me—
in many ways, they're right—

But there are times
when I feel like
crawling into a corner
like a sick cat
and just licking my wounds—

Maybe, maybe—for just a time
there's not much wrong with that.

Maude S. Newton

7

STAGES OF FAMILY ADJUSTMENT

We must find a way to accept the disease. Adjusting to the reality of Alzheimer's disease in a loved one is a complex and difficult process. Yet we must find a way to reconcile ourselves to the disease as best we can, for accepting the disease makes it easier to handle the emotional and physical strains that Alzheimer's brings. If we continue to deny the disease and its implications, we risk denying both the victim and ourselves the support and care that are needed.

Adjusting to Alzheimer's is like adjusting to a death. Because Alzheimer's is a fatal disease and one that often involves a lingering death, the stages of grief that family members go through are very similar to the stages of adjustment to death described by Dr. Elizabeth Kübler-Ross in her 1969 book, *On Death and Dying*. It is useful to understand these stages, both as they correspond to one's own psychological adjustment to the disease and for the light they may shed on the reactions of other family members.

Each individual finds her own way to become reconciled to the disease. Not everyone will go through these stages in the same way, of course, and some family members will find it easier to accept the disease than others. Each individual will probably find that she can reconcile herself to what is happening at some times better than others. Often we may misinterpret the reactions of those around us or wish they would adjust differently. If family members accept the idea that each person must face up to the disease in his own way, however, the family can serve as a strong support system throughout the adjustment process.

We must be understanding of the adjustment process of others.

In one family, for example, a mother and her son may react very differently to the illness of the father. The mother may feel a helpless anger and compensate by becoming overly involved with the illness, shutting out her son. The son may feel abandoned by his father and snubbed by his mother and may lash out in frustration when she refuses to let him help. Rather than make things more difficult for each other, both mother and son must work to understand the other's adjustment process and to accept it, as long as serious questions of sufficient care or the caregiver's health are not involved.

In considering the family's stages of acceptance, it is important to remember the following facts.

- Each family member must have the chance to work through the stages of grief to final acceptance of the disease. This does not mean that encouragement and support are not needed, nor that professional help is not indicated.

- What family members are willing to do about the loved one's needs and their own is influenced by where they are in the adjustment process. Caregiving is not simply a mechanical experience; it also involves one's thoughts and feelings.

- The adjustment process does not always occur in clearly defined stages. Long-standing conflicts and repressed feelings may need resolving before acceptance can be reached. In such cases, professional counseling may be advisable.

Kübler-Ross' stages of acceptance

The following are Dr. Kübler-Ross' stages of adjustment to death.

1. Denial and isolation. The person experiences shocked disbelief when faced with imminent death. She thinks: "No, this can't happen to me . . . it can't be true!"

2. **Anger and resentment.** The person's thoughts revolve around "Why me?" and "What have I done to deserve this?" She feels anger and bitterness toward others, the world, and even herself.

3. **Bargaining.** In her mind, the person tries to buy back her life with some promise or action. "I'll do anything if you'll give me another day, a year, five years," she may think. God may be called on in the bargaining to heal the person and restore life.

4. **Depression.** The person despairingly gives in to death because it cannot be stopped. "What's the use?" she thinks. "Why go on fighting?"

5. **Acceptance.** The person withdraws into peace and a final rest.

While these reactions are generally experienced by the dying person, family members may experience them as well.

The stages defined by Kübler-Ross do not entail all that is involved in one's acceptance of death. Some persons may never accept death. They may die still angry that life has cheated them. A spouse may be depressed for months after the death and remain angry even longer.

Perception of loss is an individual experience.

It is not appropriate to compare one family's loss with the losses of others. However, some families may be affected by the following factors that make their loss especially difficult to accept.

1. **The age of the person when Alzheimer's is diagnosed.** Younger victims forced to leave their jobs must contend with loss of income and insurance benefits. The healthy spouse may still be working, which makes arranging for caregiving more difficult.

2. **The general health of the victim.** When the Alzheimer's victim is in otherwise good health, the feeling of being cheated by life may be more intense. A person may have been prepared for cancer or heart disease but not a mysterious illness like Alzheimer's.

3. The length of the illness. The emotional strains of extended caregiving, along with its physical and financial costs, may intensify the family's feeling of abandonment and loss.

4. The family's expectations. Alzheimer's disease may be nothing like the family imagined, or the family may feel disappointed in the response of health professionals to their loved one's condition.

5. The family's emotional closeness. The afflicted person's loss of social and intellectual capabilities creates tremendous barriers to communication, and some families may not be able to counteract their sense of separation and isolation from the person.

6. Preexisting family roles. The spouse affected by Alzheimer's may have been responsible for managing most, if not all, of the family's affairs. The manifestations of the illness create a greater threat to the spouse-caregiver when she must assume the new duties of family management plus caregiving.

Adjustment to the disease usually includes five stages. The following stages of family adjustment are based upon the stages identified by Kübler-Ross but have been modified by Paul Teusink and Susan Mahler (see Bibliography) to reflect the normal series of responses that families go through when confronted by Alzheimer's disease.

1. **Denial.** Reflects the initial response that nothing is wrong.

2. **Overinvolvement.** Similar to bargaining; represents an attempt to compensate for the illness and associated impairments.

3. **Anger.** Follows when the family realizes that compensation has failed.

4. **Guilt.** Develops out of the anger and "what ifs" precipitated by looking back.

5. **Acceptance.** Resolution or acceptance of the problems.

Each of these stages will be treated in depth.

1. Denial

**Denial is
a natural
reaction.**

Denial is the most common and frequently used defense, and it comes into play from the beginning. Beliefs about senility and old age lead the family to excuse the victim's forgetfulness and thus help to sustain denial. Family members really may not feel certain that anything serious is wrong.

**Denial can
create
dangerous
situations.**

Denying the problem allows family members to postpone action. When the person lives alone, children may resist evaluating what is happening. Neighbors or friends may call to report some concerns; children may visit the parent to check these reports. However, their own denial prevents them from doing more than visiting more frequently or encouraging the parent to get out and do more.

The denial also prevents the family from adequately recognizing or facing the extent of the impairment and its consequences. The family's failure to understand such consequences places the loved one in a higher risk situation, particularly if she is living alone.

**Denial can
create family
conflict.**

Some family members may recognize that action needs to be taken but encounter denial from other family members. If a family leader is denying the problem, it can be more difficult for the others to get professional help for the affected relative.

Denying symptoms is a normal defense against threats to one's well-being. It is normal and necessary to gradually adjust to the implications of the disease. The slow progression of the illness provides time for the family to make this adjustment and to accept what is happening.

**Denial creates
barriers to
care and
family
involvement.**

Excessive denial can be quite destructive, however. It blocks help and any movement toward acceptance. Plans for care cannot be made until a realistic assessment of the patient's and the family's needs is made.

Moving past denial

The following steps will help families to move past denial:

- Seeking and receiving information about Alzheimer's disease and the family experience

- Getting a professional evaluation of the victim's degree of impairment

- Understanding the consequences of the impairment and, with professional assistance, becoming sensitive to the patient's reactions to the illness

- Seeking counseling with a professional if denial is excessive

- Addressing issues emerging from the denial with personal, family, and professional support.

A thorough evaluation of the patient's condition involves numerous health professionals.

During the actual evaluation process, it is quite appropriate for families to seek a second opinion. However, seeking many opinions can indicate desperate denial. In most situations, the Alzheimer's diagnosis already involves several opinions. For example, the following evaluative process is used at DePaul Center, a psychiatric hospital in Waco, Texas. Such a process addresses the need for a comprehensive evaluation to effectively plan activities involving the patient, family, and community resources.

Medical evaluation. Includes basic tests (e.g., blood chemistry, chest Xray, electrocardiogram, etc.) and specified elective tests (e.g., EEG or brain scan). Additionally, a neurologist or other specialists may be consulted.

Psychiatric evaluation. Assesses the presence of other psychiatric illnesses consistent with symptoms, such as severe depression; considers medications' effects and utilization as well as other medical findings.

Social history. Includes psychosocial history and assessment of the family system, resources available, and resources needed.

Psychological/Neuropsychological testing. Assists in differentiating strengths and weaknesses related to dementia and a person's emotional reactions to it; identifies actual deficits related to impaired brain function or other psychiatric disorders.

Therapy evaluation. A physical therapist and occupational therapist evaluate functioning and determine rehabilitation needs and potential.

Even when family members seem to accept the diagnosis of Alzheimer's disease, denial may leave them vulnerable to shopping for cures or believing that medication prescribed to manage symptoms will cure the disease.

False hopes Sometimes, denial reemerges when there seem to be fluctuations in the person's condition. Good days seem to promise the person is improving. Bad days intensify the family's worries that the person is deteriorating rapidly. Families can profit most by getting off the emotional roller coaster of alternating hope and despair, while making the most of the good days.

2. Overinvolvement

Stage two of the family reaction is overinvolvement. The primary caregiver may try to meet every need of the affected person, become severely isolated, and refuse assistance or support from any source. Often, the individual demonstrating overinvolvement is a spouse, although families as a whole can be overinvolved as well.

Overinvolve- Once family members overcome the denial stage
ment seeks to and admit to themselves that the illness exists,
counter the they naturally want to take action. For the fam-
impact of ily of an Alzheimer's patient, active involvement
the illness. with the victim represents a way to attempt to counteract the effects of the illness and compensate for their relative's losses. The impact of the

illness can be made less noticeable when the family is covering for the relative in all areas.

Overinvolvement can spur families into action. A family's overinvolvement can become a tool for providing the best possible care to the afflicted relative. As this stage begins, the family can plan their involvement in the overall care. Particular attention should be paid to support for the Alzheimer's victim and her spouse, who very likely will become overinvolved. Overinvolvement is a form of bargaining. When compensations fail, other strong emotions emerge.

Overinvolvement can create barriers to asking for help. Overinvolvement becomes dangerous, however, when it reaches extreme proportions. Many persons who become overinvolved fail to seek help when they should. Loyalty, duty, family, and cultural values, combined with a strong sense of obligation, reinforce the view that the caregiver must handle the illness alone. Nonetheless, such individuals reach a point when they are more open to help, even though they may not ask for it directly.

Extreme overinvolvement can lead to greater isolation and to the caregiver's sacrificing herself to the illness. Examples of caregivers who have experienced major health problems, such as high blood pressure and stress-related illnesses, are common.

Help for the overinvolved caregiver The following is an outline to follow in helping the overinvolved caregiver.

- Explore and discuss available options. A caregiver may accept the need for help in the home before she can consider institutionalization.

- Involve other family members and friends in different aspects of the care situation.

- Help the caregiver to relinquish the burden of guilt by pointing out that the patient's needs have surpassed the resources of any one person.

- If true, emphasize that the type of care needed cannot successfully be provided in the home setting.

- Help the caregiver to realize that her overinvolvement is hurting both the patient and herself, and is likely creating problems for the rest of the family.

- Suggest that lessening the spouse's care load may improve the quality of time she spends with the loved one.

3. Anger

The third stage of the acceptance process is anger, which can stem from the added physical and emotional burden caused by continued deterioration in the person and the caregiving situation. The caregiver's dedication and sacrifices may not seem to have made any difference. Also, the resources needed may not be available or may cost more than the family can afford.

Angry reactions cause guilt. Caregivers who have been tolerant of their relative's embarrassing behavior may begin to get angry as the behavior moves beyond their control. In turn, the loss of control may precipitate guilt feelings. Unfortunately, some family members lose even more control under intense stress and verbally and/or physically abuse the loved one.

Anger can stem from feelings of abandonment. The family can feel angry about being abandoned by the clearly dysfunctional relative, which can be further complicated by long-standing interpersonal problems. Whether justified or not, a caregiver may be hostile toward family and friends. Feelings of being left alone and having to make all the decisions by oneself can intensify anger. However, angry outbursts should be avoided, as they can alienate family members from one another. The anger stage of acceptance may leave the primary caregiver and others in the family quite sensitive to critical remarks about the care decisions they have made.

Misdirected anger is common. While a person is in the anger stage, her reactions can touch others who have been less directly involved with in-home caregiving. Staff members in long-term care facilities need to recognize that anger is a part of the road to acceptance. However, family members should recognize and address its real source. Otherwise, it can be misdirected toward persons who are crucial to the loved one's care or others who play vital roles in supporting the family.

4. Guilt

Guilt is a normal reaction to Alzheimer's. However, those involved must take care that the powerful combination of unresolved anger and guilt they feel does not become overwhelming and develop into serious depression. (See Chapter 3.) Caregivers may need professional help to resolve unrelenting feelings of anger and guilt.

Guilt can arise from old conflicts. Much guilt can arise from family conflicts left unresolved over the years. Family members may dwell on past regrets, wishing they could only do things over. Relatives may find themselves dwelling on such questions as "What if an evaluation had been done a year sooner?" or "What if we had seen another doctor?" They may think "We should have done more for her and spent more time with her while she was healthy." But the family must eventually put aside such thoughts, forgive themselves, and go on living.

Guilt about the wish for death It is not uncommon for family members to wish that their loved one would die and then feel guilty about that wish. As hard as it is to lose someone, most persons can view death in the last stage of Alzheimer's disease as a real blessing for their loved one and for those who cared so much for so long.

**Regrets can
become over-
whelming.**

Guilt also can be triggered by the caregiver's angry acts or imagined omissions. Perhaps she did
not do enough, or perhaps she lashed out at her
relative in frustration. But the caregiver must not
let regrets and guilt overwhelm her; it is only human to occasionally lose control under such
stressful circumstances.

**Other sources
of guilt**

Family members often find themselves giving
their relative with Alzheimer's information that is
not completely true. They may tell their relative
they are taking her to the store, when the destina-
tion is really the doctor's office. They may not be truthful about the
purpose of a medication for delusions or agitation. These "white lies"
are sometimes a source of guilt because family members believe they
are being dishonest with their loved one, tricking her or lying to her.
It is best to remember the motivations behind these actions.

**Half-truths and
caring**

Half-truths may be necessary for appropriate
care or to help families manage their affected relatives. Persons with Alzheimer's disease fail to
understand the logic behind many actions as
their illness progresses. Attempts to reason with them will only make
matters worse in many cases. If they become extremely agitated and
resistant, taking medication or trips to the doctor can become major
caregiving stressors. Family members need not feel guilty about
many of the half-truths they use to care for their loved ones.

**Tough deci-
sions can
create guilt.**

Decisions made against the wishes of the patient
can leave the caregiver struggling with feelings of
guilt. If a spouse or child forced the visit to the
doctor, she may feel guilt after the evaluation
confirming the diagnosis of Alzheimer's. Likewise, placing her loved
one in a nursing home or another institution can raise doubts and
feelings of guilt. Hopefully, this conflict can be handled by realizing
that the loved one's needs cannot be provided for at home. Most

likely, the caregiver already has done all she could and given much more of herself than she would have thought possible.

5.   Acceptance

The fight is over.   Acceptance, the final stage of a family's response to Alzheimer's disease, is possible when the process of the disease and its effect on others is fully understood. It is easier once the family members have found within themselves the resources to cope with Alzheimer's. Resources in the community become a part of their strength and are accepted in turn once they fully comprehend the impact of the illness.

The anger and guilt associated with each person's adjustment is now behind her, and she can see each stage's place in moving toward a more peaceful acceptance of fate. She can recognize, without reservation, that her loved one is no longer the person she once knew.

New situations can precipitate a return or regression to earlier stages of adjustment. The need to let go of unfinished plans or dreams, or the comments of friends and family may trigger a temporary setback. The caregiver should understand that such experiences are simply brief detours, rather than roadblocks in the adjustment process.

8

VALUES, BELIEFS, AND THE CAREGIVER EXPERIENCE

Expectations influence our feelings and reactions. It is not an easy job to change our expectations or image of a person we have known for years. However, an examination of our beliefs about the Alzheimer victim's behavior can give caregivers new insights into interacting with loved ones. Using this revised perspective, the caregiver can gain more control of the situation and can help the person with Alzheimer's to retain his capacity to reason, understand, and act appropriately as long as possible.

Taking forgetfulness personally What the caregiver believes about the Alzheimer's victim and behavior definitely influences what he feels and how he reacts. If he believes the loved one is asking the same questions over and over just to annoy him and thus becomes irritated, this irritation will be obvious to the Alzheimer's victim, even though he probably will not understand what he has done to annoy the caregiver. Such needless irritation is stressful for the caregiver, and it can have an emotionally unsettling effect on the Alzheimer's victim, leading to other, more complicated problems. It is therefore important that each caregiver learns not to take the victim's behavior personally.

Unrealistic expectations can lead to anger and frustration. A caregiver's expectations of himself also affect how he cares for a loved one. Many caregivers put great pressure on themselves. Lacking a full understanding of the physical causes of the illness and its impact on the victim's functional capabilities, they hold themselves responsible for their relative's problems and failures. Anger, guilt, frustration, and similar feelings push the caregiver beyond his limits. Caregivers must realistically assess their limitations plus the resources available. Otherwise, the stress of caregiving can lead to desperation and fatigue.

Previous adjustments to illness and loss can predict our adjustment to Alzheimer's.

Caregivers must learn to solicit and accept the help of others during the course of the illness. Those of us who find this difficult should examine our beliefs. Do we believe it is our sole responsibility to provide for all the person's needs, or is it a responsibility to be shared by other family members? Also to be considered is how well we tend to take care of ourselves. In the past, have we become so consumed by the needs of our family and others that we neglected our own needs? In the caregiving role, how are we responding to the needs of our loved one? What beliefs do we have about our role? These questions are critical to the basic pattern of our caregiving.

The caregiver should allow the patient to remain as independent as possible.

As the disease progresses, the caregiver will find himself shouldering increased responsibility for the patient. In particular, a child may find himself caring for a parent with Alzheimer's in ways that the parent once cared for him. This phenomenon is known as role reversal. It is very important, however, not to speed up this reversal process any sooner than is absolutely necessary. Alzheimer's disease is a gradually progressive illness, which means that a person does not lose all capabilities suddenly and simultaneously, nor does his family need to take over his total care all at once. The caregiver can best help the Alzheimer's patient by allowing him to remain as independent as possible for as long as possible. When the person providing care attempts to take control over all areas of the person's life simultaneously, some very unfortunate consequences such as the following may result.

- The person refuses to admit he needs any help at all and rejects all aid.
- The adult relationship between the caregiver and the afflicted person is severed prematurely.

- The self-concept of the Alzheimer's victim is eroded by doubts about his existing abilities.
- The person with Alzheimer's becomes prematurely dependent.
- The caregiver becomes overwhelmed by the unnecessary burden created.

Caregivers must therefore monitor themselves to make sure that, in their desire to be helpful, they do not hasten the end of the loved one's self-sufficient life.

Changes are not always obvious. On the other hand, family members may overlook symptoms of the disease and therefore fail to provide aid soon enough. If contact with the person is only occasional, they may have no reason to suspect that a medical condition is responsible for subtle changes in the person's grooming, dress, speech, or behavior.

It is normal to minimize changes in a loved one. When changes occur, particularly in a spouse, we tend to ignore them, if possible, or to attribute changes to temporary circumstances. It is often easier to dismiss things that irritate or bother us than it is to deal with them, especially when they do not seem to be cause for alarm. If the spouse continues to have problems, we may still feel hesitant to get a professional opinion.

Each member of the family adjusts differently. If the severity of the problems is more apparent to some family members than to others, conflict may arise among them about the best course of action. For example, Betty may want to play down her husband John's increasing problems with memory and suspicious ideas. When her son and daughter insist that she take their father to a doctor, Betty may deny that a problem exists, leading her son and daughter to become as distressed by their mother's behavior as by their father's. Betty is in conflict; her denial suggests she is having trouble thinking about the frightening possibilities. Additionally, there is the issue of convincing John to see a professional about problems he blames on her and others. Betty may believe that the family holds her responsible for what her husband is doing and what might be happening to him.

Examining beliefs helps caregivers respond more constructively to problems. It is natural at times to have counterproductive reactions to the problems of Alzheimer's disease. It can be a very difficult balancing act to determine what caregivers can and cannot expect, how much assistance should be offered, and how much is too much. The point is that caregivers should not blame themselves or their loved one, but examine how their beliefs influence their thinking, the way they act and react, and the emotions they experience and express. Such a self-examination will help caregivers to respond more constructively as they begin to care for a family member who is affected by a disease that significantly changes his behavior and character before it changes his health.

A case study shows how beliefs influence actions. The following personalized example will help to illustrate how a caregiver's beliefs can influence his reactions to a typical problem arising from a spouse's Alzheimer's condition.

Problem: Helen is yelling at her husband Tom. From the bedroom she screams, "Come here! You never come fast enough when I need you!" Then she bursts into tears.

Belief: Tom believes that his wife Helen depends on him too much and should do more for herself. He knows she has Alzheimer's, but he feels she is being lazy. He has always felt she was a demanding person. When he hears her crying, he thinks to himself that it is just like her to get hysterical about nothing.

What beliefs relate to Tom's thoughts and feelings? Because he thinks Helen is just being lazy, Tom feels aggravated. This feeling grows as he considers how often she depends on him to do things that she really could do for herself. He is already washing dishes, which is not his job. Her crying irritates him more than it frightens or concerns him; he believes she cries to get what she wants. Because he feels manipulated, he becomes angrier.

Tom's reaction: "Helen, shut up! I'll be there in a minute, or you can come in here." Tom is too angry to ask her what she needs or to go to the bedroom immediately. He disregards the fact that his wife now has difficulties in clearly expressing her needs.

Helen's problem: Actually, Helen has slipped out of the chair in her bedroom. She is not hurt, but she is frightened and upset. She has made statements in the past about her husband not coming to her when she asked, even before the Alzheimer's condition, and that almost habitual response has slipped out when, in a panic, she cannot describe what has really happened. The disease has affected her coordination, and in her fright, she cannot organize her movements to pull herself up. She is crying out of fear and frustration.

Tom is reluctant to respond to the initial yelling because of past experiences. He still does not understand the impact of the illness well enough to appreciate how it is eroding his wife's ability to manage for herself. Neither does he appreciate the insecurity created by the illness.

With a clearer understanding of Helen's limitations, Tom might ask her if something is wrong or simply walk into the bedroom. He has probably gotten tired of taking care of his wife and feels frustration and anger. These negative reactions toward his wife are intensified by his feelings of being unappreciated. His irritation has delayed his response to Helen, who is sitting on the floor unable to get up, feeling frightened and upset.

Caregivers can respond more appropriately to problems when they identify the various reasons for their reactions. The previous illustration shows that the perceived problem is not always the real problem, and that beliefs and feelings about a problem can lead to interpretations, judgments, and reactions which can prevent caregivers from successfully handling the problem.

ACCEPTANCE

You have Alzheimer's disease
and you're losing the power
to remember—to reason—to understand,
to do the simple tasks
we take for granted:
to put on a shoe—
to button a shirt—
to read a book—
to remember a face or name.

It's a hard thing to understand—
to accept . . . .
Perhaps it's been the hardest for me,
for I've lived with you—
but I know—you can't help it—
can't act otherwise . . . .

I must take you as you are
and expect—not more—but less
as the disease continues to progress.

Maude S. Newton

9

HOW TO RESPOND POSITIVELY TO ALZHEIMER'S BEHAVIORS

In Chapter 2, we discussed the symptoms of Alzheimer's disease. Even when we recognize a disturbing behavior on the part of our loved one as an Alzheimer's symptom, however, it is not always easy to know what the appropriate response should be. Unaccustomed to our loved one's new impairment, we naturally tend to respond to the behavior as we would have in the past when the person was healthy. Unfortunately, this often means responding with annoyance, frustration, and anger—which, as we have seen, is not helpful either for us or the Alzheimer's victim.

This chapter suggests more productive ways to respond to common disturbing behaviors exhibited by Alzheimer's patients. After listing the behavior, we first identify the common immediate reactions. Usually this is an interpretation and response that would be appropriate if we were responding to a healthy person's behavior, but it is not a useful response to behavior by an Alzheimer's patient. We then guide the reader through a better interpretation of the behavior, one based on an understanding of the brain impairment produced by Alzheimer's disease. Finally, we offer specific suggestions for productive ways of responding to the problem.

Our goal is to create an accurate and practical guide to caring for Alzheimer's patients that will help both caregivers and patients enjoy the good days and minimize the bad days. Our examples cannot possibly cover all situations. However, when caregivers learn this approach, they can use it with different situations and in different care settings.

Behavior	*1. The person asks the same questions over and over.*

Common Responses

The person is not listening or trying to remember; she wants attention or is trying to annoy you; she should be able to control this.

Alzheimer's Interpretation

The person is suffering memory loss, which in turn creates a strong sense of insecurity and uncertainty. She may be asking the same questions repeatedly because she seeks reassurance and security, or perhaps your earlier answers seemed vague or unclear. She may sense you are avoiding the answer, which could heighten her sense of insecurity.

In more advanced stages, memory impairment may be so severe that she does not recall asking the question, or she may feel threatened by your earlier answer. For example, if she asks repeatedly when she is going to the doctor, the doctor may be a source of insecurity for her.

Helpful Responses

- Respond clearly, slowly, and concretely to questions.
- Have the person repeat what you have said.
- If you suspect that your earlier answer disturbed the person, provide reassurance and/or factual information that will set her mind at rest.
- Distract the person into other activity or other topics of discussion and ignore further questions.
- Avoid arguing or responding with anger; do not rebuke the person for the memory problem.
- Write down the information in question for the person who can still read.

Behavior	*2. The person's personality appears to have changed.*

Common Responses	She is going crazy or having a nervous break-down; she has lost all self-respect and pride.
Alzheimer's Interpretation	Personality changes are characteristic symptoms of Alzheimer's. Often, these changes are observed prior to any clear impairment of memory or intellectual abilities. Brain impairment associated

with Alzheimer's can radically change the way the person acts. Additionally, personality characteristics can be exaggerated in early phases of the illness.

Subtle changes in personality can represent an early signal that a problem exists. If the person realizes that she is acting in ways which are not like her, she may fear that she is having a nervous breakdown or losing her mind.

Eventually the brain impairment erases most traits of individuality. Some examples of personality changes follow:

Normal Personality	*New Traits*
Socially active	Socially withdrawn
Calm, easygoing	Worried, easily upset
Kind, understanding	Selfish, demanding
Relaxed	Paranoid
Emotionally controlled	Excessively emotional
Careful, cautious	Careless
Good judgment	Poor judgment
Sexually sensitive	Sexually demanding
Friendly	Unfriendly, hostile
Honest	Dishonest
Flexible	Rigid
Loving	Uncaring

Helpful Responses

- Accept personality changes as results of, or reactions to, brain impairment.
- Try to satisfy the needs underlying behavior, such as the person's need for security, self-esteem, dignity, and love.

Behavior	*3. The person does not do what she says she will or leaves a task uncompleted.*
Common Responses	She is lazy and not really trying; she is lying to you; she wants your help with everything.
Alzheimer's Interpretation	Memory impairment makes it more difficult to do something that was agreed upon. For example, seeing a shirt laid on the bed may no longer trigger the idea that the person should put it on.

Memory abilities cannot be separated from intellectual abilities, such as reasoning, and both faculties are being lost.

Helpful Responses

- Use reminders and memory lists.
- Maintain a routine for daily activities.
- Make requests close to the time the task is to be completed.
- Provide step-by-step assistance for more complicated tasks.
- Always request the desired behavior in the same setting (e.g. eating in kitchen or dining room, dressing in bedroom or bathroom).
- Provide verbal assistance if the person seems to have forgotten how to complete parts of the task or has forgotten what she is doing.

Behavior	*4. The person denies her memory problems and makes excuses for mistakes, blames others, or seems unaware of the problem.*
Common Responses	The person is not being honest; she should face the problem and accept responsibility for her own mistakes; she is just getting old and senile.
Alzheimer's Interpretation	Denial of memory problems is a very common response to Alzheimer's. Initially, denial is a necessary defense. It protects the person from

frightening changes that are difficult to accept. If she makes excuses or blames others, she may be desperately trying to explain the memory impairment without directly confronting the problem.

Helpful Responses

- Avoid forcing the person to face up to the memory problems.
- Provide reminders or suggest checklists as ways to aid memory.
- Be understanding of the threat that memory impairment poses for your relative.
- Arrange for the person to talk to a professional if she seems troubled but cannot admit the problem to her family.

Behavior

5. The person insists she does not need help because she has always done things for herself; she becomes angry when you offer assistance.

Common Responses

She is stubborn and unreasonable; she is rejecting you personally; her anger is unfair.

Alzheimer's Interpretation

The person's refusal of help is an effort to maintain independence. Anger directed toward you may really be caused by her frustration with the illness. Her self-worth and self-esteem are threatened. Later, such denial may show she has lost a grasp of her own needs and problems.

Helpful Responses

- Determine what help is needed and provide what is needed in a kind manner.
- Realize that the person may genuinely lack awareness of her needs and problems.
- Provide encouragement and reinforcement for even the smallest successes and for acceptance of your help.
- Avoid overemphasizing the person's weaknesses or communicating disgust.

- Avoid confronting problems too directly if you suspect the confrontation could provoke strong emotional reactions.

Behavior	*6. A spouse's sexual interests and demands are higher than normal or more difficult for you to satisfy.*
Common Responses	A sexual relationship is inappropriate in light of the illness. How could she enjoy sexual activity at such a time?
Alzheimer's Interpretation	Brain damage can increase a person's desire for sexual activity. It also can decrease her sexual inhibitions, create difficulties in relating sexually, and reduce sensitivity to her partner. Alzheimer's

can threaten a person's sexual identity and self-esteem.

The loss of intimacy that occurs as the disease gradually diminishes the victim's personality may make it difficult for the caregiver to sustain a sexual relationship. The affected person may continue to find sexual satisfaction, but the spouse suffers a loss of emotional satisfaction.

Despite these problems, sexual relations can continue to be important, and they are a matter of personal choice. The person with Alzheimer's needs to feel wanted and loved. Adjustments in relating sexually may be necessary.

Helpful Responses

- Understand changing sexual interests and demands in the context of both the illness and your prior sexual relationship.
- Rely upon touching, being caressed, and nonverbal relating as substitutes for the sex act.
- Talk with a physician or counselor if the sexual problems persist.

Behavior	*7. The person mishandles her money and monthly bills; she accuses you and others of stealing her*

money; she claims her banker is handling money matters.

Common Responses

She is inconsiderate and irresponsible; she is unfair and will not face the facts; she is lying and avoiding the issue.

Alzheimer's Interpretation

Having and handling money is one of the symbols of a person's independence and competence. The person may blame others for her mistakes because she is trying to protect her self-esteem and maintain her independence.

Early problems with memory and reasoning abilities make it difficult to handle more complex financial matters. Trying to perform calculations, even on paper, becomes frustrating. Accusing others of taking money is one way in which the person fills the gaps in her memory and protects her self-esteem.

Helpful Responses

- Be sure there is no truth to accusations of theft, particularly when the person lives alone and is vulnerable.
- Let the spouse or adult child assume the responsibility for financial matters.
- Monitor the person's monthly bills and contact creditors about questionable charges.
- Be sensitive to the person's insecurity and fears when discussing financial matters.
- Allow the person to have some cash on hand to enable an easier adjustment to alternative financial arrangements.
- Consider legal arrangements such as power of attorney and guardianship as means of protecting the person's financial security.

Behavior

8. The person tells ridiculous stories or says unusual things.

Common Responses	She is lying or being mean; she is going crazy or getting senile.
Alzheimer's Interpretation	Such stories are easy to take personally, but they are rarely malicious. As memory and reasoning abilities continue to decline, larger gaps are left in the person's perception of reality.

It is harder for her to explain or understand what is happening because her grasp of logic is deteriorating. Ridiculous stories and obvious untruths may be attempts to fill in the blanks, to explain what she cannot understand.

If the person believes her own stories, the things she says may cause real agitation, anger, and fearfulness. If her stories place blame on others, she may be trying to defend her self-respect and integrity.

Some of the unusual things a person says may also represent difficulties in speech. Finding words to explain things or even name things correctly becomes difficult as the disease develops. The person may be able to manage only fragmentary ideas or statements.

Helpful Responses

- Clarify and correct the person's understanding of events.
- Respond sensitively to underlying feelings of insecurity, fear, or frustration.
- Avoid overreacting to stories or allowing an argument to start.
- Distract the person with conversation about other things.
- If the person is upset, give her a chance to calm down.

Behavior	*9. The person wants things to be done immediately; she wants you to do everything.*
Common Responses	The person is being inconsiderate; she is acting childish and overly dependent; she is attempting to control you.
Alzheimer's Interpretation	If the person was demanding before the brain impairment, the disease could accentuate such traits. In addition, her loss of memory may have

triggered anxiety and panic, and her demanding or overly dependent behavior may be an attempt to gain control. Her anger may mask fear.

Helpful
Responses

- Remind yourself that there is no point in becoming frustrated and angry.
- Respond calmly.
- Let the person know what is going on and being done.
- Do something with the person, even if not what is being asked.
- Talk to other people about your feelings, frustrations.

Behavior

10. The person repeatedly talks about experiences from the past.

Common
Responses

She is living in the past; she does not want to relate to the present.

Alzheimer's
Interpretation

Although the brain-impaired person's ability to recall recent experiences is becoming less reliable, she still may remember more remote material from the past. This material remains accessible to the person longer and can provide a more meaningful basis for self-esteem and identity. The present has become more threatening and difficult to accept emotionally. The person may also be losing her ability to relate to time and may be confused about the relation of past to present.

Helpful
Responses

- Use past memories to make activities in the present more meaningful.
- Provide concrete information that distinguishes the present from the past; for example, contrast pictures of grown-up grandchildren with their childhood pictures.

- Set aside time for reminiscing.
- Patiently and supportively orient the person to the present when confusion is apparent.

Behavior	*11. The person's abilities fluctuate from day to day or hour to hour; she remembers some things but not others.*
Common Responses	She remembers what she wants to; she is not trying to remember; she must be getting old and senile.
Alzheimer's Interpretation	It is normal for the memory of all Alzheimer's patients to fluctuate in this fashion. It is a mistake to believe that improved memory on a given day means the condition is improving, however.

Some information or events may be easier to remember. Material that is unpleasant or threatening may be more easily forgotten.

Helpful Responses

- Make the most of good days.
- Determine the kinds of information more easily recalled.
- Note if a certain manner of presenting information improves some kinds of memory.
- Realize that the person will tend to remember more under relaxed and quiet circumstances.

Behavior	*12. The person continues to drive the car despite safety problems.*
Common Responses	She is being stubborn and showing poor judgment; she should give up driving.
Alzheimer's Interpretation	Driving gives a person freedom and control of her daily life. Denying she is lost or confused,

despite obvious problems, is her way of defending her self-esteem and independence. Confronting her about mistakes may produce more vigorous denial and angry reactions.

Despite resistance, family members must limit and eventually eliminate the person's driving opportunities. Even during the early stages of the illness, the person is vulnerable in situations requiring quick decisions because her reaction time is impaired. Alzheimer's also affects visual perception, including perception of distance.

Concentration difficulties will eventually erode the person's ability to drive safely. For example, if the traffic light before her changes to green but a car on the intersecting street is going through the red light, the brain-impaired person may be unable to decide which change is the most important. Too many things are happening at once, and her problem-solving abilities become overwhelmed.

Giving up driving is very difficult for most people with Alzheimer's. They may be more willing to stop driving if another health problem, such as visual impairment, is cited as the reason. Most caregivers will want a loved one to stop driving long before the affected person is ready.

Helpful Responses

- Enlist the support of other family members in convincing the person to stop driving.

- Enlist the help of the person's physician, attorney, insurance agent, mental health professional, or trusted friend; the instructions of authority figures may be followed more closely.

- Discuss the problem with your insurance representative.

- Contact your police department or department of public safety and inquire about license nonrenewal, suspension, or restrictions and other procedures to ground an unsafe driver.

- Remove keys or dismantle the car's starter as a last resort.

- Understand the person's anger and resentment about such a loss and avoid confrontations about driving difficulties.

- Remember that removal of driving responsibilities eliminates the possibility of an unfortunate accident.

Behavior	*13. The person accuses you, family, and friends of doing things or makes up stories about you.*
Common Responses	She is becoming paranoid, losing her mind, being unfair, becoming unmanageable, or trying to hurt or embarrass you; she is getting senile.
Alzheimer's Interpretation	Such problems are other ways in which brain-impaired persons react to the insecurity created by memory loss. In this case, the problem more directly involves the caregiver, since the victim is

most likely to accuse her spouse and other close family members.

Arguments tend to reinforce beliefs. Confrontations and other negative approaches tend to worsen the situation rather than help it.

Helpful Responses

- Avoid contradicting the person directly, as this may only make her angry and confused.

- Avoid highlighting mistakes and give calm and reasonable explanations; communicate a sense that things are all right or will improve.

- If something is lost, offer to help find it or suggest specific places it could be found.

Behavior	*14. The person has hallucinations or bizarre and frightening delusions.*
Common Responses	The person is mentally ill; Alzheimer's is getting worse.
Alzheimer's Interpretation	Progressive brain impairment affects an individual's ability to interpret information accurately. Hallucinations are often misinterpretations of real sights and sounds. Delusional beliefs repre-

sent an attempt to fill in gaps of information and explain what happened. For example, if the person says someone is knocking on the walls and is trying to break into her house, she may really have heard a tree branch rubbing against the house. Insecurity, so often associated with progressive brain impairment, leads the person to interpret events from a fearful and threatening perspective. Suspiciousness is a common response to a person's diminishing control of her world.

When a person seems to be talking with someone who is not present, she may not actually see or hear the person, but she may be involved in a delusional belief, such as thinking a deceased person is alive or talking to a child who lives 400 miles away.

A number of other problems contribute to hallucinations and delusional beliefs. These include medical problems such as infections, changes in diabetic conditions, or pernicious anemia. Medications also must be evaluated.

Other conditions that impair a person's ability to receive information can contribute to hallucinations or delusional beliefs. Hearing or visual impairment are examples.

Helpful Responses

- When delusions or hallucinations are observed, consult a physician.
- Provide the person with concrete information.
- Show support for the feeling of the experience, responding with reassurance.
- Avoid arguing or disagreeing with the person, as that will only upset her more.
- Try to distract the person, move her to another room, or talk about something comforting.

Behavior	*15. The person becomes disinterested and withdrawn in social situations.*
Common Responses	She does not care about friends or people anymore; she wants you to stay home all the time.
Alzheimer's Interpretation	The person's cognitive and memory deficits are making it very difficult to follow social conversations and interact appropriately. This inability

leads to frustration and anxiety in social situations, thus prompting her to withdraw.

This withdrawal may be preceded by restlessness, tension, and agitation. If the demands on the person are not decreased, she may become more upset or even rude to uninformed observers.

**Helpful
Responses**

- Provide emotional support and verbal assistance in demanding social situations and observe any obvious changes in the person's anxiety level.

- When the person becomes nervous, encourage her to simply withdraw from the social situation for a while.

- Anticipate the more demanding situations before they become uncomfortable.

- Inform friends about her behavior and how they can make her participation easier.

- Search for those social situations that are less demanding.

Behavior

16. The person is very restless, cannot stay still, or is easily agitated.

**Common
Responses**

Something is bothering her; she does not have anything to do.

**Alzheimer's
Interpretation**

As the disease progresses, agitation and restlessness commonly accompany the insecurity created by the person's diminishing abilities to cope. Denial and rationalization, which previously helped to block out awareness of functional losses, become less successful protective devices as her problems become more pronounced.

Some restlessness may suggest anxiety and underlying fears, though the person cannot always explain these feelings. Too much stimulation can contribute to anxious and agitated behavior. Medication given to control these symptoms should be carefully monitored, as it can sometimes intensify the symptoms it was prescribed to decrease.

**Helpful
Responses**

- Use a calm, reassuring approach that supports her feelings, even when the underlying source is not apparent.
- If she can say what is bothering her, try to eliminate the source of trouble; if she cannot, avoid pressing for explanations.
- Reduce noise and activity levels.
- Ask the physician if the agitation can be decreased with medication or if medication might be creating the undesired effects.
- Involve the person in an activity that helps burn off excess energy.

Behavior

17. The person constantly watches you and follows you around.

**Common
Responses**

She wants too much attention; she is overly dependent; she will not entertain herself; she is suspicious and distrustful of you.

**Alzheimer's
Interpretation**

This problem develops from the fear and insecurity caused by the person's memory impairment; watching or following the caregiver provides greater security. Such behavior also promotes her sense of belonging and alleviates her sense of isolation, which might otherwise intensify anxiety and fear.

Mistrust or suspiciousness may develop because the person is less sure of what is happening. Her interpretations of information and her reasoning capabilities are less reliable. Some persons develop paranoia or more intense suspiciousness as a response to a more threatening world outside themselves.

**Helpful
Responses**

- Understand such behaviors as a search for security.
- Identify and alleviate specific fears that are creating insecurity, for example, the fear that you are leaving the house.

- Orient her as to what is happening and clarify what you are doing.
- Spend time with the person.
- Engage her in constructive activity; ask her to do some supervised things with you.
- Avoid dramatic changes in routine.

Behavior	*18. The person's moods change for no apparent reason. She gets upset and even aggressive if cornered.*
Common Responses	The changes are related to medication, changes in her condition, or something you have done; she is losing her mind and cannot control her emotions.
Alzheimer's Interpretation	Such mood swings are often related to changes in the body and brain as the disease progresses. The mood swings also can be precipitated by thoughts and ideas the person has but is unable or unwilling to express.

The person may also be experiencing a catastrophic reaction, which means that the person is overwhelmed by too much happening too quickly, has become extremely upset by her confusion and loss of control, and cannot respond adequately to the situation.

Helpful Responses

- Consult a physician if significant mood swings occur without cause or are increasing in intensity.
- Remove the person from the upsetting situation slowly and quietly.
- Be realistic in your expectations and avoid pushing.
- Reduce outside stimulants.
- Avoid expressing anger and frustration.
- Avoid reasoning or arguing, but use nonverbal support such as holding hands in a calming fashion.

Behavior	*19. The person refuses to bathe and groom; she says she has already done so.*
Common Responses	She does not care about her personal appearance; she is being stubborn and uncooperative; she is lying.
Alzheimer's Interpretation	Regular bathing and attention to personal hygiene lose their social significance for persons with brain impairment. Social judgment and awareness diminish.

Since taking care of personal hygiene is the most basic sign of independence, however, it becomes threatening to adults to become dependent upon someone's help to bathe and groom themselves.

Bathing can become embarrassing to the brain-impaired person. Being nude, closed in, and helpless in a bathtub or shower creates a sense of vulnerability that may be frightening.

Because the person is accustomed to bathing regularly, it may make perfect sense in her mind to claim she has bathed.

Helpful Responses

- Maintain bathing and grooming at regularly scheduled times.
- Make bathing and grooming comfortable and relaxing experiences; offer, for example, a warm bath and relaxing back massage.
- Be aware of potential fears such as anxiety about falling or water that is too hot.

Behavior	*20. The person fails to recognize familiar persons, places, and things.*
Common Responses	She is getting much worse and is terribly confused.
Alzheimer's Interpretation	Due to a kind of brain impairment known as agnosia, the person is gradually losing her function of recognition. What her eyes see no longer can

be put together into the previously meaningful and understandable picture. Thus people, places, and things she has been around all of her life now truly appear unfamiliar.

**Helpful
Responses**

- Avoid arguing when this occurs, as conflict will increase the person's confusion and fear.
- Agree that things look different and calmly indicate who you are or identify the thing in question.
- Bring specific and recognizable things to the person's attention to help reestablish contact with the past.
- Avoid rushing the person.

Behavior	*21. The person wanders around at night or seems to be looking for something.*
Common Responses	She is confused and does not know what she is doing; she is being inconsiderate.
Alzheimer's Interpretation	Wandering may occur when the person is disoriented in the middle of the night and has forgotten her reason for awakening. The sleeping difficulties may be caused by frightening noises,

hallucinations, or nightmares. When there is a lack of structured daily routine, the difference between night and day is less pronounced.

**Helpful
Responses**

- Reorient the person when she is wandering in the household.
- Reassure the person that she can look for whatever she wants tomorrow, after a good night's sleep.
- Keep a light on in the bathroom.
- Consult a physician if sleeping difficulties persist.
- Increase the person's level of activity during the day.

Behavior	*22. The person refuses to eat, or she eats very little.*
Common Responses	She has a poor appetite; she is too picky about food; she needs to be more active.
Alzheimer's Interpretation	As Alzheimer's progresses, it is common for decreases in appetite to occur. Eating binges and a desire for sweets also occur, but greater concerns are created by the refusal to eat.

Often persons fail to eat because they believe they have already eaten or because they simply forget what they are doing. This is more likely to occur with persons who live alone or in situations where structured daily routine is minimal.

Brain impairment also contributes to difficulties in using eating utensils. Swallowing can be difficult.

Helpful Responses

- Minimize between-meal snacks.
- Maintain as high a level of physical activity as possible.
- Provide regular meals that follow a routine.
- Eat with the person.
- Prepare familiar and favorite foods.
- Be sure food can be easily chewed and swallowed.
- Cut meat as necessary; use utensils that are easy to hold.
- As coordination deteriorates, offer direct assistance.
- Consider using vitamins or food supplements.
- Avoid overemphasizing neat eating habits.
- Give the person more time to eat.

Behavior	*23. The person does not seem to care for you anymore, and she says you do not love or care about her.*

**Common
Responses**   She no longer loves and appreciates you.

**Alzheimer's
Interpretation**   As brain impairment progresses, the person's awareness of the people around her naturally diminishes. She becomes less expressive and makes fewer gestures of appreciation. When she questions whether you love or care about her, she may be seeking reassurance to counteract her sense that she is losing you due to her diminishing abilities.

**Helpful
Responses**

- Reassure her that you care, without taking offense at her questions.

- Provide as much involvement as possible with other individuals and supporting influences, such as an Alzheimer's Family Support Group.

Behavior   *24. The person's hands and arms shake; she stumbles and is unsteady when she walks.*

**Common
Responses**   She is nervous; she has visual problems; her arthritis is getting worse.

**Alzheimer's
Interpretation**   While nervousness may be responsible for some of the shaking, other causes also should be considered. Side effects of medications prescribed for severe agitation, delusions, hallucinations, and sleeping problems may be the source. Stiffness also could be caused by these medications.

In other cases, tremors may be directly related to the brain impairment. Rapid jerking movements of the limbs or even the body can occur. These are called myoclonic jerks and should be evaluated by a physician.

Loss of mobility and coordination of large (gross) and small (fine) movements occur with the disease. These coordination problems contribute to difficulties with all motor skills. Weakness, poor balance, and stooped posture make walking difficult; likewise, difficulty in getting up from a chair leads to long periods of sitting. Prompt medical attention should be sought as these conditions escalate.

Some persons with Alzheimer's may exhibit symptoms suggestive of Parkinson's disease. This neurological disorder can coexist with Alzheimer's, but it is difficult to differentiate when Alzheimer's is in its advanced stages.

Helpful Responses

- Check to be sure that poor vision or other impairments do not restrict the person's mobility.
- Change furniture, lighting, throw rugs, and so forth to promote safety at home.
- Provide the person with ample opportunities for exercise to prevent premature weakness and loss of coordination.
- Avoid rushing the person, provide assistance when required, and encourage her to carry out tasks one step at a time.
- Consult a physician when dramatic deterioration in motor skills occurs.

Behavior

25. The person sits doing nothing for long periods of time.

Common Responses

She should be doing something worthwhile; she should be more active; she is bored, lazy, or depressed.

Alzheimer's Interpretation

As brain impairment affects memory and intellectual abilities, spontaneous and self-initiated activity diminishes. Apathy and a lack of interest in what is going on develops because the person's ability to partake in daily life is compromised. Her abilities to plan and carry out purposeful activity are likewise affected by diminished cognitive abilities. Later, she may develop problems with walking and standing. More positively, sitting quietly may be a welcomed relief for her from the increasingly stressful demands of daily life.

**Helpful
Responses**

- Develop daily routines that include enjoyable activities which require minimal concentration.
- Encourage and assist the person's participation in shared activities.
- Walk and exercise with the person to encourage muscle strength and coordination.
- Realize the person may be enjoying the chance to relax and be free of stressful activities.
- Use music and some television to add stimulation to time spent sitting.

Behavior	*26. The person wets or soils herself.*
Common Responses	She is not trying to control her bodily functions and does not care any more; she wants your attention; she is trying to get back at you for something.
Alzheimer's Interpretation	These problems are not uncommon in more advanced stages of Alzheimer's. The person is less aware of the need to relieve herself and does not associate this need with the bathroom.

Memory problems and perceptual difficulties make it more difficult for the person to find the bathroom. At night, disorientation and confusion make it more difficult to use the bathroom.

**Helpful
Responses**

- Assist the person in maintaining regularly scheduled trips to the bathroom.
- Leave a night light on in the bathroom.
- Consider reducing the intake of liquids in the evening.
- Label the bathroom door and help the person practice finding it.

- Be understanding of bladder and bowel accidents, which are quite embarrassing to the individual.
- Have a doctor examine the person for other underlying medical problems.

Behavior	*27. The person wanders aimlessly.*
Common Responses	She is disoriented and lost; she does not have anything to do.
Alzheimer's Interpretation	Wandering is a problem for people who have brain damage. Because of the potential conse-

quences of wandering, it is a behavior with potentially dangerous outcomes. The person could fall or become lost in the neighborhood. (We have considered some aspects of wandering in *Behavior 16,* restlessness/agitation and *Behavior 21,* nocturnal confusion.)

Wandering cannot be easily understood if one sees it as aimless. In fact, what appears to be aimless wandering is not an aimless activity at all in many cases. A brain damaged by Alzheimer's disease merely has difficulty determining the purpose or goal of such activity. The impaired person may not be able to communicate; thus the caregiver cannot arrive at the reasons with questions. In such cases, the caregiver may find that the purpose of the wandering becomes clearer through observation. Often people who are thought to be wandering aimlessly follow the same path repeatedly. This may be more evident in institutional settings. Along that path are sources of positive stimulation (outside views, water, coffee, social contact). Wandering can also be an effort to avoid or escape adversive situations, such as dark or noisy areas and more isolated spots which create a strong sense of insecurity.

Other explanations for what appears to be wandering behavior include the following possibilities.

1. The person is looking for something she has lost.

2. The person does not recognize her surroundings and may be looking for something familiar. (This may be an example of agnosia—failure to recognize familiar persons, things, places— or a reaction to new or changed physical environment.)

3. The person is more confused, restless, or agitated as a reaction to tranquilizers or other medication.

4. The person may be more confused during certain parts of the day, for example, early morning or late evening.

5. The person may be confused as a result of sensory impairment. Because she hears or sees poorly, she cannot comprehend sights and sounds accurately. These types of impairments can also result from brain damage. In this case, the individual cannot process visual and auditory information correctly, and her perceptions are distorted.

6. The person may wander as a response to stress. She may walk away from upsetting situations and then become lost. A catastrophic reaction may precede the wandering behavior. Some persons may have always gotten upset easily by a stressful situation and walked away from it.

Helpful Responses

■ First, determine the type of wandering. Is it really aimless, or is the wandering goal-directed?

■ Then, determine if the wandering is an attempt to gain something (stimulation, food, drink, security, or physical activity because of restlessness).

■ Remember that restlessness and pacing are common during some phases of Alzheimer's disease. Supervise this activity constructively. Walk with the person in a safe and stimulating area. (Too much stimulation can be overwhelming at times.)

■ Determine if the wandering behavior is a response to stressful environmental factors. For example, too much noise or demands placed on the person too quickly and forcefully may precipitate behavior that results in wandering and getting lost.

■ Determine if the person's apparent wandering is a reaction to fear. Has the individual misinterpreted sights or sounds? Are these delusions or hallucinations? Is she trying to get away from something that frightens her? If so, wandering may be her attempt to seek security and safety. Relate to this need.

- At night, leave some lights on and the door to the bathroom open, so the person does not get lost on the way to the bathroom.

- If you believe the wandering is created by medications, consult your physician for a medications review.

- Place locks on outside doors that cannot be undone by the organically impaired person but which you can open easily.

- Have the person wear a MedAlert-type bracelet which says "memory impaired." A name, phone number, and address on this or some other items will also be helpful.

- If wandering continues to be difficult to manage, consult a physician or mental health professional.

Wandering is a major source of stress to most caregivers. Understandably they worry about it because of its potential harmful outcomes. Caregivers should take action to deal with this problem, or it will create more stress and heighten the need for supervision considerably. If the memory impaired person does wander away from home, notify the police department immediately. Having pictures of the person along with an accurate description of such characteristics as hair color, height, weight, and other identifiers will increase the chances of the person's being found quickly. Be sure to tell the police that the person is memory impaired, confused, and so forth. You may offer suggestions on how the person may be best approached. If you know, tell police about the status of the person when she left. Was the person upset and angry? It may be better for the caregiver to remain home and have family or friends assist with the search so that someone is at the home should the patient return there.

When the person returns home, it will be better to relate positively to the return. Your anger or scolding will only make matters worse. The person will probably be frightened anyway.

ENIGMA

Isn't it strange . . .
That which we have long perceived
as a burden—
the care of a sick loved one—
the care that went on
and on and on—is over now?

It was tiring, and confining,
and discouraging and demeaning at times.
Yet—in a strange way—
I can feel no relief.

Perhaps, inadvertently,
he gave my life a purpose—
a purpose I hardly recognized
nor appreciated.

Now I need a new purpose
(and I am old for that).
That covenant has been kept
as best I knew how—
But my life goes on.

Help me to find a new purpose—
a new resolve—
and let it be a life that doesn't
just keep on living.

Maude S. Newton

10

EXPLORING COMMUNITY RESOURCES

Some communities have better resources than others. Since the early 1980s, Alzheimer's disease has received considerable public attention. The media has given particular emphasis to the impact this illness has on both its victims and their families. Nonetheless, most communities do not have services and care facilities developed specifically for the long-term needs of Alzheimer's patients. Nor do they provide support services for the family; for example, not all communities have sufficient day and respite programs which address the needs of both patient and caregiver. However, most communities do have agencies that provide for the various long-term care needs of the elderly, and these agencies often provide support and service to Alzheimer's patients and caregivers.

Drawing upon community resources reduces strain on the caregiver. Throughout this book, the importance of calling upon community resources has been stressed. In this chapter, the creative and appropriate use of these resources will be discussed in more detail. Such resources can allow the family to care for the Alzheimer's victim at home without a severely restrictive quality of life. The caregiver has been described as the hidden victim of this illness, and his needs cannot be ignored. But the physical and mental strain placed on the caregiver can be significantly reduced if both family and community resources are sufficiently utilized.

Families need to plan ahead and to explore community resources before the need becomes critical. Family members may feel at first that they prefer to manage alone. But community resources become more important as the primary caregiver grows more isolated and fatigued. Interest in exploring other resources naturally develops as the caregiver begins to wonder how much longer he can continue in the caregiver role. A need for outside help will also surface as the patient's deterioration produces greater difficulties in management and self-care. It is therefore advisable that families explore the resources available in their communities in the early stages of the disease, so they are prepared when the eventual need for more help arises. Families equipped with facts about what lies ahead find it easier to anticipate and plan for the future.

Finding out about helpful services The first step in utilizing community resources is to identify what resources exist. The following are some good places to begin when searching for the resources in your community.

- *Health Professionals.* Family physicians, psychiatrists, mental health professionals, social workers, and others already involved with the Alzheimer's patient are a natural starting point. Ask them for referrals and resource suggestions to address the needs and problems at hand.

- *Community Mental Health Centers.* Mental health centers that have services for the elderly or offer more specialized Alzheimer's care can be a valuable information resource. These agencies can work with the person who has Alzheimer's and his family or spouse. After determining the types of resources needed, the agency can link families with the services that exist in the community.

- *Area Agencies on Aging.* These agencies are involved in developing community resources supportive of the needs of the aging population. Persons with Alzheimer's represent a special part of this population, and area agencies on aging are likely to be knowledgeable about local resources that will support Alzheimer's care.

- *Medical Information and Referral Programs.* These programs exist to aid persons seeking information about and help with medical conditions of all kinds. They may be attached to a governmental agency, a care facility, or a program for the elderly. To locate such a program in your community, contact a medical facility or the Agency on Aging.

- *Alzheimer's Resource and Information Centers.* More recently, some communities have developed programs that specifically address the resource and informational needs of the Alzheimer's patient and family. Such programs may survey the individuals' needs and help caregivers manage their situations. They also may refer the family to other community social-service or mental-health programs developed for the aged or persons with Alzheimer's.

- *Alzheimer's Family Support Groups.* These groups provide important information about more formal local resources that support the care of the Alzheimer's patient. Such groups also may provide information about individuals who can be hired to stay with the person in the home and help with personal care and supervision.

Developing goals for caregiving   Once the family knows the full range of resources available, members can choose the ones most helpful in their situation. In determining how to use resources, the family may wish to reflect on the goals of caregiving. Often, the overall goal of caregiving is to keep the relative in the familiar surroundings of his home. However, refining this goal can provide the caregiver with more definite guidelines for selecting community resources. He should draw upon those that can help him to:

1. *Maintain the patient's social and self-care abilities at the highest possible level.* Premature dependencies place an excessive strain on the family caregiver. To maintain the person's abilities, an appropriate degree of social activity and stimulation is needed, which the family cannot always provide.

2. *Support the patient's adjustment to the gradual losses and limitations associated with the illness.* Persons with Alzheimer's can benefit from supportive counseling, particularly in the

disease's earlier stages, and they can appreciate emotional support for their adjustment throughout. Opportunities for the patient to continue in familiar activities with some degree of success are needed. These successes help support the patient's self-esteem and offset other losses that occur.

3. *Support the family's adjustment to the degenerative process of the disease and the stresses of care.* Family members may need supportive counseling to come to grips with the illness and to learn to work supportively with one another. The ongoing activity of caregiving must be supported to avoid the emotional and physical breakdown associated with stress.

4. *Maintain the safest and most supportive environment.* Basic needs must be provided for, and the person must be safe from danger, neglect, abuse, or exploitation. These concerns particularly apply to persons who live alone.

5. *Provide relief from the constant responsibility of caregiving.* Relief from constant supervision of the person, for example, may be possible when a nurse aide assists a few hours a day with personal care and housekeeping. Caregivers can use outside resources to care for their relative, providing opportunities to take care of their own needs.

Guidelines for using resources

Community resources are meant to support, not replace family involvement. In relying on community services, family members should follow these guidelines.

- Ask questions to clarify your understanding of the situation.
- Express your own needs and concerns.
- Use contact with one community resource as an opportunity to learn about other resources that might be helpful.
- Seek information provided from community resources and professionals when making difficult decisions.

Some community resources that are helpful in caring for Alzheimer's are discussed in the following section. The "Service/Resource" worksheet has been included in the appendix for caregivers to use in comparing and selecting resources.

Community Resources for Alzheimer's Care

1. *Alzheimer's Family Support Groups.* These groups provide caregivers with support in coping with the illness and in dealing with problems experienced in caregiving. Self-support groups also can be a source of information about the disease and community resources. Participants experience similar problems and assist each other in making decisions about care. The emotional adjustment of the family to the illness is promoted by such groups.

2. *Respite Care.* This type of service provides family members with occasional relief from the pressures of continuous caregiving. Such relief can prevent premature institutionalization of the patient as a result of the caregiver's physical and emotional stress. Formal respite programs offer services ranging from several hours' to several weeks' relief.

   Respite care also occurs when families hire persons to relieve them from duties in the home. Some families are able to take turns caregiving. In other situations, respite comes as a secondary benefit of medical or psychiatric hospitalizations.

3. *Shared Respite Care.* A number of families with Alzheimer's victims may join together to provide caregiving on a rotating basis. Typically, several family members watch over a group of patients to allow others to have some free time. Benefits are experienced as the Alzheimer's patient and spouse participate with other patients and their families in an activity setting outside the household. By caring for their loved one in company with others, caregivers find that social isolation is reduced. The burden of providing activities becomes an opportunity that is shared by participants.

4. *Adult Day Care.* Some day programs are designed specifically for persons with Alzheimer's. Others provide structured activities to a more heterogeneous group of impaired older persons or other age groups. Day care provides exercise, activities, recreation, support of daily living skills, counseling, and monitoring of the participant's general health. Such programs can help the person with Alzheimer's maintain some abilities that would otherwise deteriorate more quickly. Some provide more specialized social work, nursing, or physical and occupational therapy services. By utilizing adult day care, family members can remain employed, do errands, rest, and be involved in other important areas of their lives.

5. *Home Health Care.* Home health programs usually can provide nursing and personal care services to patients in their homes. For persons with Alzheimer's disease, nursing care is usually not needed until the later stages of the illness, unless other coexisting medical problems exist. But supervision and personal care are very important needs of the Alzheimer's patient. Many home health programs have nurse aids, homemakers, or care providers that can assist with these needs. Self-employed persons also can be hired to provide supervision and assist with the person's personal care needs. Persons with Alzheimer's will definitely need this type of care when they live alone and have no family who live nearby. Home health personnel can help with a broad array of supervisory and direct care needs such as meals and shopping, medications, cleaning and washing, transportation, appraisal of the person's condition, and companionship.

6. *Legal Services.* Often family members must consider questions such as the person's ability to handle finances and make decisions for himself. Protection of the person and property must be considered, but not at the expense of his other rights and privileges. Alzheimer's disease does not automatically make a person incompetent. When some form of legal guardianship is being considered, the opinion of the treating physician, a psychiatrist, or other mental health professional should be solicited prior to legal consultation.

7. *Community Mental Health Centers.* Some community mental health centers have specialized geriatric programs that can be very helpful in the management of the Alzheimer's client and supportive of the family caregiver. These programs can provide a wide range of services, including comprehensive assessment, psychiatric evaluations, individual, group, and family counseling. Additionally, case-management services identify other community resources that can help with home maintenance. Referrals can be made and service linkages developed.

Some persons with Alzheimer's disease may present serious behavior management problems. Even when such problems are not apparent, however, the caregiver may find mental health centers helpful in planning care.

Mental health intervention may help in cases of an especially lengthy period of caregiving, a patient with difficult personality traits, a difficult living environment, or other large-scale problems.

Among the specific behaviors that indicate a need for immediate attention are the following:

- Hallucinations and delusions that contribute to sleeping disturbances, agitated and combative behavior, or disruptive interactions with neighbors and community.
- Severe confusion and disorientation.
- Physically threatening behavior.
- Harmful resistance to necessary care and management.
- Potentially dangerous activities such as wandering, driving, and so forth that the family cannot stop.
- Depressive symptoms early in the course of the illness.
- Anxiety, agitation, or denial so extreme that they make care management difficult.

Needs that can be addressed by a mental health center's case-management services include:

- Severe lack of family support.
- High level of caregiver stress.
- An inadequate caregiving situation, such as that of a person who lives alone.

8. *Psychiatric Hospitals.*   Private psychiatric hospitals offer assessment and behavior stabilization. They may be the best resort in cases of unmanageable behavior. The hospital staff can often assist the family with care planning and management.

Considerations for Nursing Home Care

Reevaluating appropriateness of in-home care   Families can use other resources to maintain the loved one in the home. However, conditions may develop that require family members to reexamine the appropriateness of in-home care. Usually these conditions are beyond one's control. Professionals can assist families in deciding whether to place the person with Alzheimer's disease in a nursing home. The following questions should be considered.

1. Can the total needs of the loved one be adequately provided for on a 24-hour basis in the home?

2. Has the health status of the individual changed so that more nursing care and medical monitoring are necessary?

3. Is the stamina of the caregiver severely taxed by the care situation in the home?

4. If the person lives alone, is there adequate supervision and assistance available to provide for his needs on an ongoing basis?

5. Is it realistic to expect the family to deliver or purchase the services the relative now needs in the home?

6. Are the financial resources of the spouse becoming severely threatened?

7. Do health concerns for the caregiver begin to rival those for the Alzheimer's patient?

8. Has the caregiver's isolation become severe?

9. Is the in-home care contributing to the emotional/physical breakdown of the caregiver/spouse?

10. Is the nursing home placement as unacceptable as it first seemed?

11. Will the quality of contact with the Alzheimer's victim improve by placement in a nursing home?

12. Will the family be able to pull closer together around the nursing home placement?

13. Have physicians and other professionals recommended such a placement?

14. Have the caregiver's approaches to daily problems become ineffective?

Dementia is common in nursing homes. Nursing homes are becoming more aware of the needs of the Alzheimer's patient and the family. Nursing homes have been dealing with this illness disguised by other names for a very long time, and a high percentage of the persons in nursing homes has some form of dementia or cognitive impairment.

Determine whether the Alzheimer's unit provides special services.   Some nursing homes have developed Alzheimer's units to more adequately address the total care needs of these individuals, and others are considering such approaches. Special Alzheimer's programs can provide a more meaningful role for family members. However, families must determine whether such units actually provide specialized services rather than just grouping the patients together.

When choosing a nursing home for a relative with Alzheimer's disease, families should consider several factors.

1. Is the staff physician familiar with Alzheimer's?
2. Are staff at all levels of the nursing home aware of the needs and problems associated with this disease (e.g., administrative, nursing, dietary, and activities staff)?
3. How do staff interact with residents who are similarly impaired?
4. What activities are provided for persons with Alzheimer's and other dementias?
5. Is the physical plant of the facility well organized, attractive, and designed to encourage either socialization or privacy as appropriate?
6. Does the facility encourage family involvement and support groups?
7. Is the atmosphere friendly?
8. What provisions are made to prevent wandering?
9. Is the building particularly noisy?
10. Is there a safe area for the person to walk outside?
11. How does the facility deal with residents who are noisy and hard to manage?
12. How are drugs and restraints used in behavior management?

13. Is the facility a reasonable distance from your home?

14. Do Alzheimer's units utilize a special approach to needs of these residents?

Some families may realize that a nursing home may be the most appropriate resource for the care of their relatives with Alzheimer's disease. Still, they may have built barriers to seeking the placement. Some concerns are practical, others psychological. The following example illustrates some psychological barriers that should be overcome.

Suzy was the middle-aged daughter of a 75-year-old man who had Alzheimer's disease. Suzy was the primary caregiver because her two brothers lived out of town. Her relationship with her father had not been particularly close. However, she shouldered the responsibility for his care, partly because she felt guilty about her past with her family. She had been divorced for ten years, and during that time she had assumed a major role in caring for her parents. She still believed her brothers should help more, but their explanations for not being more involved generally were reasonable. They did help somewhat with financial needs. Her mother had died a year before in a nursing home. Now her father was living with her.

The mother had a strong role in caring for Suzy's father until she had suffered a stroke, which eventually precipitated her placement in the nursing home. At that time, the father had objected to his wife's leaving. Suzy thought he had been angry with her since that time; certainly he was more agitated. Suzy had visited her mother in the nursing home, taking her father along. These visits had often upset her father. He would accuse her of trying to put him away.

Now the father required more care and supervision. Suzy still felt some guilt about the past, but she experienced new feelings of guilt about her mother's placement and how she thought it had affected her father. She was experiencing more guilt in caring for her father. It was painful to Suzy when he asked for his wife or called Suzy by his wife's name. One night he talked frequently about going home. Suzy did her best to assure him he was home, but in his state of agitation, he would not listen. Later that night he wandered from the house.

Suzy's father was not found until the early morning hours by the police, who took him to a hospital emergency room. Suzy was awakened by a call after her name and number were found in his billfold. Her dad was so confused and agitated that he had to be placed in a psychiatric hospital for a few days.

The father responded well to that setting, yet it appeared to the hospital staff that he needed more care than Suzy could provide at home. Nursing home placement was recommended, but Suzy insisted that she must care for him at home. For a while her position seemed unreasonable to staff until the past and current sources of guilt were uncovered. Suzy actually believed she could provide better care in her home, particularly now that her dad was more stable.

Hospital staff agreed to support this decision if Suzy would get help from some community services to help her manage her father and deal with her needs. Counseling eventually helped Suzy to accept her limitations in caring for her father. She finally reconciled her feelings of guilt to the extent that she was willing to look at some other nursing homes. She had gotten involved in the Alzheimer's Family Support Group whose members helped her look at some facilities better equipped to care for Alzheimer's patients and to involve family members in constructive ways. Suzy also involved her brothers in the decision, so she did not have to feel it was her decision alone.

Three months later the placement was made. After a month, Suzy was confident they had made the right decision when she saw her father doing a little better than he had at home. She became involved in some of the nursing home's activities and maintained a modified caregiving role with her father. She began to have a life of her own again.

Finances can be a real barrier to nursing home care. Financial arrangements can be a practical barrier to nursing home placements even when families desire placement. Public assistance programs for nursing homes, such as Medicaid, have financial requirements that must be fulfilled before the cost is covered by a mixture of state and federal funding. Family members should investigate this resource long before their relative needs nursing home care. Too often nursing home placement is sought in a crisis. A hospital may be about to discharge the person, or the caregiver may either have become too ill or too overwhelmed to continue to provide care himself.

In many states—Texas for one—there are two types of eligibility that must be met before nursing home placement can be covered by state and federal financial resources: financial and medical. This can be confusing to families. Not only are there two types of eligibility, but there are also two different state departments that approve the two types of eligibility. Since Alzheimer's disease is not yet uniformly considered a medical condition, there may be problems in getting medical eligibility established. The deficits in the person's functioning must be almost overemphasized for the person to qualify as having medical and nursing care needs. The treating physician may not be familiar with all aspects of daily functioning and mental status. (Forms in the appendix should be helpful in establishing the degree of impairment.)

Families may need to elicit help from attorneys and other agencies in establishing financial and medical eligibility. Private pay does not require such planning, but many people with Alzheimer's disease cannot afford private pay at all. Contact with nursing homes may help families seeking nursing home placement if they start making their plans early. Agencies involved in establishing eligibility should be contacted to determine what information is required. Steps in that process should be fully understood by families. As a rule, if families are familiar with eligibility requirements and the process involved in nursing home care, the eventual placement will take place more smoothly. Early planning also enables family members, particularly the spouse who remains at home, a chance to plan for financial security.

Some patients with Alzheimer's disease may be eligible for other long-term care services, such as placement at a Veteran's Administration (VA) hospital or nursing home care unit. This too should be investigated so that family expectations can be based on facts and not assumptions. The placement may not be possible because the veteran does not meet eligibility requirements. Others who meet requirements may not stay in the VA system for long-term care. The VA also contracts with community nursing homes for placement.

Final Resource Considerations

Family members caring for a relative with Alzheimer's disease usually have more resources and services available to them than they utilize. Long-term care in the home is possible. In some cases care can be provided in the home until the relative's death. Planning care will involve the need for strategic utilization of community resources, other family members, and friends. Services for Alzheimer's care vary from one community to the next. Rural areas and small towns usually have fewer services than urban areas.

Costs for services also vary. Some have state, federal, and local funding. Others are funded by foundations and other grant sources. Still others are private and require full payment unless other arrangements can be made. Insurance may cover some services, but at this point family members should not assume too much about insurance coverage. They should investigate what types of care and services insurance will cover and for how long. Some families face a difficult predicament when they assume insurance covers nursing home care. While policies may cover some nursing home care, long term care is not usually covered.

Few communities have sufficient and affordable resources for Alzheimer's care, particularly day care alternatives and respite care services. Other services may be unavailable or simply inadequate to meet the ongoing needs of in-home care. Many provider-type programs that supply in-home services such as cleaning and personal care cannot accept responsibility for supervision. The hours a week that such services can be provided are often limited. In-home supervision is, nevertheless, a major need. On a short-term basis, in-home respite care or a brief respite placement can be beneficial.

Persons living alone and suspected of having an Alzheimer's-type condition are quite difficult to help when family is absent or nonexistent. In these cases some type of guardianship or protective services may be necessary to provide care. Unfortunately, many communities do not have guardianship programs where a nonrelative guardian can be appointed. Mental health authorities may be able to help if these persons reach a point where they are a danger to themselves or others. However, even then the long range plans may have no solutions.

Family caregivers are a source of ideas for what services are needed in their communities. In fact, families feel less helpless in these situations when they find a way to bring needs to the attention of agencies and others who develop programs in the community. One of the better options is to contact an Area Agency on Aging, which is charged with the responsibility of identifying needs of the elderly, planning for those needs, implementing, and monitoring programs funded under the Older Americans Act. (See the list of these agencies in the appendix.) There may also be other community agencies which are active in planning and program development. The Area Agency on Aging may be able to direct caregivers to these other resources in the community.

PART II
RESEARCH AND TREATMENT

In this part of the book, we have dealt with the more technical aspects of Alzheimer's disease, first describing the physiology of the brain and the changes that take place, then discussing treatment possibilities, keeping in mind that developments are happening daily. Finally, we describe medications typically used and possible side effects.

Survivors

For years I've watched
an old mesquite tree—
gnarled and bent and twisted—
buffeted by winds and droughts.

It starts to grow up
toward the sun and sky.
But the soil is so poor,
the water so scarce,
the heat so fierce,
so cold at times,
it was beat to the ground.

Each Winter you'd think,
—It's dead, for sure!
It's succumbed to the odds
stacked against it.

Yet wait 'til the Spring
and a miracle occurs,
New life springs up
from the gnarled old branches—
a tiny chartreuse sprout
heads straight for the sun!
It lives—overcoming
all that is hard,
telling all the world,
—I live, I will survive!

Sometimes I feel like that old mesquite tree
I feel battered by life's adversities,
I feel down—but not out!
When Spring rolls around,
I feel a fresh stirring of life.

I have things to do—
places I want to explore,
people I love!
I can hold my head high—
look the world in the eye—
and say,
—I live, I will survive!

Maude S. Newton

11

ABNORMAL CHANGES IN
THE BRAIN

For hundreds of years, the symptoms of what we now know as Alzheimer's disease were attributed to senility and old age, or perhaps in more recent times they were attributed to hardening of the arteries and psychosis. In the past, people feared that one day just because they were old, they would "go crazy," lose their memory, and become completely helpless without ever knowing why. With the identification of Alzheimer's disease, however, it has become possible to properly diagnose persons suffering from this illness and to at least partially alleviate their suffering. The next step, at which medical researchers currently are at work, is to isolate the exact biological causes of the disease. Once these causes are known, we can begin to develop effective treatments for Alzheimer's and perhaps someday even find a complete cure.

The next two chapters of this book offer a look at the research done to date on both the causes and treatment of Alzheimer's. This research has revealed physical and chemical changes present in brains affected by Alzheimer's, suggested possible causes of the disease, and included experiments with promising treatments.

Because the research completed leaves many questions unanswered, most of the material covered here must remain somewhat speculative. Although a great deal has been learned to date, no definitive answer to the mysteries posed by Alzheimer's disease has been found. The research findings are valuable, however, because they allow caregivers to understand more fully the changes occurring within the Alzheimer's patient. In addition, the very real progress made gives hope that someday—we all hope soon—medical research will lead us to a clear-cut strategy for the disease's treatment and prevention.

The final chapter covers the use of current medications used in treating some of the psychiatric manifestations of Alzheimer's disease. Agitation, anxiety, delusions, and sleeping difficulties present behavior management problems to family caregivers. Careful use of psychiatric medications can make caregiving much easier.

Physical Changes in the Brain

Abnormalities are found in the brains of Alzheimer's patients.

When a person is diagnosed as having Alzheimer's disease, the brain has already deteriorated to some degree. Almost without exception, physical abnormalities (such as neurofibrillary tangles, neuritic plaques, and others) are present in the cerebral cortex, the outer layer of the brain that governs such higher functions as memory, thinking, and reasoning.

Several of the abnormal characteristics of brains affected by Alzheimer's disease are associated with the most basic and important part of the brain, the neurons (also called nerve cells). The brain consists of many billions of neurons, which are its means of receiving and sending messages. Neurons can be viewed as the way different parts of the brain communicate with each other and the rest of the body. One neuron of the brain may communicate with as many as 1000 other neurons although these units of communication usually send messages to only a few neurons. Alzheimer's disease is somehow responsible for a loss of neurons. Some of the physical abnormalities, for example, neurofibrillary tangles, occur in the body of neurons. These changes might contribute to destruction of nerve cells or compromise their functioning.

Connection between disease and abnormalities

Because the tangles, plaques, and other physical abnormalities so consistently accompany the disease, researchers feel certain that some connection exists between these brain abnormalities and the mental and emotional changes that Alzheimer's patients experience. What is not well known is whether these physical changes are directly related to the cause of Alzheimer's disease or whether other aspects of the disease itself cause the abnormalities. In the latter, the physical changes would be manifestations of the illness. These are questions future research will continue to address.

Connections between abnormalities and impairments   We do know that a direct correlation exists between the degree and the distribution of physical abnormalities and the severity of Alzheimer's-type dementia. We also know that the abnormalities discussed in this chapter tend to be concentrated in areas of the brain that control abilities most affected by Alzheimer's. These findings suggest that physical changes in the brain make some contribution to the disease's impairments.

Anatomy of the Brain

To understand how Alzheimer's affects the brain, we first must understand the basics of brain anatomy and the ways in which various areas of the brain are related to specific mental functions.

Brain's cortex   The outer surface of the brain is known as the cerebral cortex (see Figure 1). Accounting for about 80 percent of total brain mass, the cortex is divided into two nearly symmetrical hemispheres: the left and the right. Each of these hemispheres is divided in turn into four lobes: the frontal, the parietal, the temporal, and the occipital.

Frontal lobes   The frontal lobes mediate motor functions, govern emotional behavior, help organize sequential physical movements, determine some abilities of expressive speech, and influence personalities, inhibitions, and social behavior. As Alzheimer's disease affects this area of the brain, patients undergo a variety of personality changes, lose inhibitions, and become less able to organize behavior. With damage to the frontal lobes of the brain, persons do not recognize their errors.

Parietal lobes   The parietal lobes are concerned with sensory functions such as physical sensations, touch, and spatial relationships. They also allow us to recog-

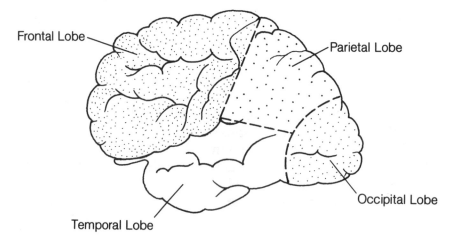

Figure 1. The Cerebral Cortex. The lobes of the brain's cortex. The frontal lobe is at the front of the head. This is a side view of the left hemisphere. The right hemisphere is basically a mirror reflection of the left hemisphere.

nize patterns in our experience, perform intellectual tasks such as mathematics, and maintain our physical orientation. Disorientation to places can result from damage to this brain area. When Alzheimer's strikes the parietal lobes, patients experience trouble with coordinated, purposeful movements, spatial perceptions, and recognition, among other functions.

Occipital lobes The occipital lobes are the brain's visual center, controlling very basic visual perceptions and bringing together the parts of visual information into a meaningful whole. Damage to this area can lead to loss of the visual field and problems in space perception.

Temporal lobes The temporal lobes are involved in a range of important functions, including hearing, memory, vision, and verbal comprehension. In conjunction with the brain's limbic system, these lobes also affect the experience and memory of emotions such as fear, jealousy, anger, or happiness. Our sense of time and individuality also seems to be located in these

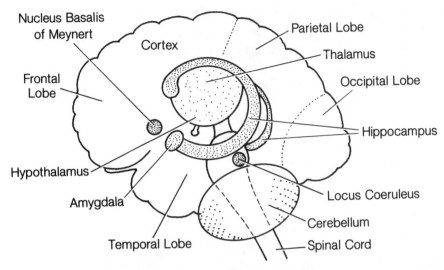

Figure 2.   Brain Areas Affected by Alzheimer's Disease.   This picture of the brain shows areas impacted by Alzheimer's disease abnormalities. The location of the nucleus Basalis of Meynert is an approximation. Other parts of the brain have been omitted because they are not relevant to our discussion. Some parts of the limbic system—the hippocampus, amydala, thalamus, and hypothalamus—are indicated.

lobes (Restak 1984). Of the four brain areas, the temporal lobes appear to be the area most severely affected by Alzheimer's disease. Memory problems, auditory perception, musical perception, difficulties in comprehension, and difficulties in execution of speech all appear to be connected with damage in this area. Problems in focused attention also can be attributed to damage in the temporal lobes.

The limbic system of the brain affects memory and emotions.

Enveloped by the cortex are a number of other brain areas relevant to an understanding of Alzheimer's disease. Some of these are part of the limbic system, a group of brain structures which have influence on our emotions and behavior. The parts of the limbic system most involved in the damage associated with Alzheimer's disease include the amygdala, believed to affect emotion, and the hippocampus, believed to affect both short-term and long-term memory (see Figure 2).

The importance of the parts of the brain just described will become clear as we further explore the physical changes that Alzheimer's brings. The reader should note that the temporal, parietal, and frontal lobes of the cortex are more affected by physical changes. The hippocampus seems to be a prime target for physical abnormalities.

Neurofibrillary Tangles

Tangles are clumps of ordinary filaments in the brain that have become abnormally twisted.

Among the symptoms of the disease identified by Alois Alzheimer in his original diagnosis in the early 1900s was the presence in the brain of something called neurofibrillary tangles (see Figure 3). Simply put, neurofibrillary tangles are bundles of ordinary brain filaments that have become badly twisted. When such tangles are viewed under an electron microscope, one can see little hair-like structures called filaments. When these filaments occur in pairs, they are wrapped around each other in a spiral fashion (Reisberg 1981), somewhat like two pieces of yarn that have been twisted together and then stretched tightly. These paired filaments are known as paired helical filaments, a term sometimes used to refer to neurofibrillary tangles. Filaments are normal; they become abnormal when their form is changed by twisting.

Figure 3.   Neurofibrillary Tangles and Paired Helical Filaments.   If the image of tangles to the left were enlarged, lines would take the appearance of the paired helical filaments to the right.

All older people develop some tangles in those parts of the brain that affect memory and behavior.

Interestingly, some degree of neurofibrillary tangle formation is found in virtually all examined brain tissue of persons over age 90 (Reisberg 1981). Tangles also are found in specific brain areas of most normal middle-aged and older persons. When their brain tissue is examined microscopically, tangle formations are particularly evident in the hippocampus, the area that plays a role in both recent memory functions and the storage and retrieval of long-term memory (Beaumont 1983). It has some involvement in learning. The hippocampus further seems to be involved in bringing together various forms of incoming sensory information (Bloom et al. 1985), the inhibition of responses, the organization of movement, and spatial organization (Kolb and Whishaw 1980). Another area where concentrations of tangles are found is the amygdala, which has a role in fear reactions and aggressive behavior. It is also suspected of having some role in memory with the hippocampus. The reader will recall that both of these structures are part of the brain's limbic system, which has a major role in expression and experience of emotion (Kolb and Whishaw 1980).

The more severe problems with memory and behavior associated with Alzheimer's may be caused by more severe problems with tangles.

Since aging persons tend to exhibit a high incidence of tangles in brain areas associated with memory as well as memory problems, it seems possible that the development of slight short-term memory loss with age could be associated with subtle damage to the hippocampus. It further follows that the more severe memory disorders of Alzheimer's patients as well as related problems might be associated with more severe hippocampal damage. Similarly, the lack of emotional response to memory problems found early in Alzheimer's, sometimes called a blunted or flat effect, could be associated with damage to the amygdala, while damage to the overall limbic system could account for patients' loss of emotional control. Altogether, the damage caused by tangles to these parts of the brain could be responsible for some of the emotional disturbances and personality changes exhibited by Alzheimer's victims.

Because tangles appear to occur naturally with age, the mere presence of tangles in the brain does not indicate disease. What is different about the brains of Alzheimer's patients, however, is the location and number of tangles. In Alzheimer's victims, tangles tend to be significantly concentrated in the hippocampus and in far higher numbers than in the brains of normal aging persons. They also are concentrated in the cerebral cortex, particularly in the parietal-temporal region and the association cortex. The association areas of the cortex bring together information from the areas around which they are located. It is in these areas that the brain integrates immediate sensory information with memories and emotions, thus making it possible for us to think, decide, and plan behavior. Since such integrated thought typically becomes difficult for Alzheimer's patients, the damage observed in the association cortex seems particularly significant.

Other small but important areas of the brain are affected by neurofibrillary tangles. These small areas represent collections of nerve cells that serve as stimulation centers for neurons ascending into the brain's cortex. Neurons or brain cells of the brain comprise an intricate network through which information can be transmitted and received.

Groups of neurons within the brain's network are specifically adapted to communicate with their own chemical messenger which is called a neurotransmitter. These special networks of neurotransmitters, specific nerve cells, each receive stimulation from their own collection of nerve cells deeper in the brain. For example, for the neurotransmitter acetylcholine which is deficient in the Alzheimer's brain, the source of stimulation is called the nucleus basalis of Meynert (see Figure 2). This brain area has a significant concentration of tangles.

Tangles are also found in the localized areas of the brain that act as stimulation centers for neurons using the neurotransmitters norepinephrine, serotonin, and dopamine (Bondareff 1986). Chemical changes in the brain are discussed later in this chapter.

Research has shown that the larger the number of tangles found in Alzheimer's patients, the greater the degree of dementia.

The correlations discovered make it likely that tangles are directly linked to the impairment of brain function, though research has not yet uncovered precisely what that link might be. Some research suggests that tangles may have some role in neuronal deterioration and destruction. The loss of neurons may also be secondary to other unknown aspects of the disease process. Other research has shown that the larger the number of tangles found, along with another abnormality known as senile plaques, the higher is the degree of dementia observed in Alzheimer's victims. This further confirms the suspicion that tangles and plaques may be a source of the disease's impairments.

Other dementing illnesses are also associated with tangles.

As an interesting sidelight, neurofibrillary tangles also have been found in other types of dementing illnesses. Among these are dementia pugilistica (punch-drunkenness), a dementia observed in veteran boxers; the rare Parkinsonian-dementia complex of Guam (Reisberg 1981); post-encephalitic Parkinson's disease (Bondareff 1986); and other forms of infectious dementias. Another disorder in which tangles are very frequently present is Down's syndrome, the genetic abnormality that causes mental retardation. Persons with Down's syndrome who live past age 40 invariably develop tangles, plaques, and other pathological changes common to Alzheimer's disease (Katzmann 1986), and the tangles are similarly located in the brain (Reisberg 1981).

Current research on neurofibrillary tangles focuses on unlocking the composition and abnormal protein source of the paired helical filaments. This is important because the protein in paired helical filaments is not common to the brain. Some researchers suggest that since the protein might come from a source external to the brain, an unconventional virus may be implicated (Selkoe 1987). Paired helical filaments have also been found in neuritic plaques. Further investigation of the paired helical filaments may lead to other clues to the cause(s) of Alzheimer's disease because they have not been found in the brains of neurologically normal persons (Davies and Wolozin 1987). By learning more about tangles, it is hoped that we will also uncover significant answers about the causes of Alzheimer's disease.

Senile or Neuritic Plaques

Significance of plaques

Like neurofibrillary tangles, plaques were among the physical abnormalities noticed by Alois Alzheimer in his original diagnosis of the disease. As with tangles, plaques are found in the brains of normal aged persons; however, they appear in far more significant concentrations in the brains of Alzheimer's victims, appear in those parts of the brain that are most affected by the disease, and are most prevalent in the most severely affected individuals. In fact, plaques appear to be an even better indicator of the degree of dementia than do neurofibrillary tangles.

Types of plaques and description

There are three types of plaques: primitive, classical, and amyloid. Classical and amyloid plaques both contain more amyloid. All types of plaques can be found in Alzheimer's disease. In classical plaques the amyloid is contained by the core; amyloid plaques consist almost entirely of this amyloid material (Wisniewski 1983). The classical plaque is easier to picture (see Figure 4). There is the central core of amyloid that appears fuzzy and fibrous. This core is surrounded by a ring of degenerating fragments of cells which resemble a loosely-arranged crown of thorns. The fragments are like the debris of brain cells and include axons, dendrites, and slender filaments. Paired helical filaments of neurofibrillary tangles can be found in the debris around the classical plaque's core. Neuritic or senile plaques are the more general terms used for the three types of plaques.

Plaques are found outside neurons, whereas neurofibrillary tangles are found in neurons. In Alzheimer's disease, plaques are abnormal, particularly because they occur more frequently than in the brains of normal aged persons. Plaques also occur in other diseases of the brain.

Locations of plaques

As with tangles, plaques tend to be more abundant in the cerebral cortex and are found in smaller numbers in other parts of the brain such as the thalamus. Rarely, they have been found in

Figure 4. Classical Neuritic Plaque. The primitive plaque consists mainly of the clustered debris outside the core of this plaque. Amyloid plaques consist of the core material of the plaque.

the cerebellum (Bondareff 1986). The thalamus receives sensory information and has some control of our motor activity. It helps us be generally aware of touch, temperature, and pain. The cerebellum primarily coordinates muscular activity and receives information from other parts of the body such as skin, muscles, and joints.

Some indication of damage to the thalamus may be observed during the course of Alzheimer's disease. Damage associated with the cerebellum would be more difficult to observe until perhaps the later stages of the illness. Functions assigned to the hippocampus and cortex are more easily recognized and more severely disturbed. Memory impairment and disturbances in thinking, judgment, and speech are common features of Alzheimer's disease.

Amyloid and plaques   With regard to this disease, the significance of plaques rests not only on their concentration in areas of the brain that are most impaired, but the presence of amyloid is also important. Amyloid is a part of the plaques, and research has shown enduring interest in amyloid because it is thought that understanding this abnormal protein might yield clues to Alzheimer's cause. Amyloid is a starch-like protein. It tends to be produced and deposited in tissues during certain disease processes.

Amyloid and disease   Amyloid has been associated with a variety of diseases that include tuberculosis, Hodgkin's disease, and cancer. Such severe neurological illnesses as Creutzfeldt-Jakob disease and Kuru are associated with accumulations of amyloid. Both are caused by slow viruses.

Amyloid and the immune system

Amyloid is known to be deposited in tissues which experience altered immunity (Thienhaus et al. 1985). For some reason, the body's immune system does not protect the body from disease effectively. The possibility is raised that Alzheimer's disease might result from breakdown in the body's immune system. Instead of protecting the brain, the immune system turns on the brain. This suggests an autoimmune response whereby the body produces antibodies that are directed against its own healthy tissue. The immune system cannot tell the difference between normal and foreign substances.

Amyloid and prions

The understanding of amyloid has been advanced some by the work of Prusiner and his coworkers. Amyloid plaques were found in a slow virus disease (scrapie) in sheep and goats. This disease has been transmitted to a hamster brain. The brain tissue was found to contain very small rod-shaped particles called prions. Prions are protein-like infectious particles (Goldsmith 1984) which are smaller than a virus. In a certain configuration prions have a remarkable resemblance to amyloid plaques, causing some researchers to hope that amyloid plaques may be found to be associated with prions. This would provide some evidence that a similar slow virus might cause Alzheimer's disease. However, the amyloid plaque in this disease could also be formed from proteins other than prions. The issue of what causes amyloid in plaques has not been settled.

Down's syndrome

The significance of neuritic plaques has been examined from another perspective. The amyloid proteins found in Alzheimer's disease are thought to be the same amyloid present in Down's syndrome (Davies and Wolozin 1987). In the Down's syndrome brain, neuritic plaques containing amyloid (as well as other abnormalities associated with Alzheimer's) typically appear in abundance and are distributed in much the same way as in Alzheimer's disease. Down's syndrome is characterized by extra copies of Chromosome 21 and is a genetic disorder.

Chromosome 21 and Alzheimer's

In 1987 some significant findings occurred involving Chromosome 21 and Alzheimer's disease. An abnormal gene on this chromosome shows a genetic defect that is thought to be responsible for a familial form of Alzheimer's disease. This indicates that some cases of Alzheimer's disease are under genetic control. This same chromosome contains a gene that is responsible for producing a major protein component of amyloid. This may be the amyloid that collects in the walls of blood vessels and/or plaques in both older individuals with Down's syndrome and persons with Alzheimer's disease.

Amyloid in Down's syndrome

The gene for brain amyloid can account for more amyloid in the Down's syndrome brain. Since there are extra copies of Chromosome 21 in this disorder, there would be more copies of the gene influencing the production of amyloid. This line of reasoning, however, cannot explain amyloid in Alzheimer's disease because there is no duplication of the amyloid gene.

Amyloid mystery

Aging itself may be a factor. As we age, amyloid may be produced. This could explain why Alzheimer's disease increases in older persons. We know that amyloid is present in the walls of cerebral vessels of aged persons (Wisniewski 1978). However, even with these deposits of amyloid, plaques do not necessarily occur. It is not clear if vascular amyloid, which is fairly common in both Alzheimer's disease and old age, has the same origin and chemical composition as the amyloid in plaques. Amyloid's presence in plaques remains a puzzle.

Amyloid near cause of Alzheimer's

At present, we only know that amyloid plays a central role in Alzheimer's disease. We do not know how. It may very well be closely connected either with the cause of Alzheimer's disease or with other underlying conditions that will lead to the cause. Since it now appears that every person has a gene that plays a part in the production of amyloid, we must question why everyone does not get Alzheimer's disease. Researchers suspect that some other factor or factors must combine with the amyloid gene's role in order for Alzheimer's disease to develop. These factors might be a virus, some chemical extraneous to the brain or body, immune system breakdown, or factors that simply have not been identified.

Amyloid involved in several abnormalities
Amyloid in plaques common in Alzheimer's disease raises many questions for research. Our understanding of amyloid is growing. It is associated with plaques, tangles, and cerebral vessels. We also know that the brain's loss of neurons corresponds with the distribution of plaques and tangles. Tangles and plaques particularly are indicators of the severity of dementia. The greater the concentration of plaques, the greater is the impairment of brain function. We cannot yet say that plaques cause the loss of brain cells.

Future research and amyloid
Amyloid may act with other as yet unidentified factors in Alzheimer's disease which accelerate the production of amyloid. As a result of this, interaction in offensive proteins may be changed into harmful deposits of amyloids. Science may be able to discover ways to frustrate the genetic production of amyloid. Other factors must be identified that can explain why everyone who has an amyloid gene does not develop Alzheimer's disease.

Granulovacuolar Degeneration

Description of GVD
A third type of brain abnormality, granulovacuolar degeneration (GVD), has an attraction to neurons in the hippocampus of the Alzheimer's brain. GVD strikes the area of brain cells around their nucleus (see Figure 5), the area called cytoplasm. One or more fluid-filled spaces, vacuoles, form in the cell's cytoplasm with GVD. Within the vacuoles there is a dense, granular material (Ball 1983) which under an electron microscope appears to have a crystalline structure (Conley 1987). As these granulovacuoles develop, they

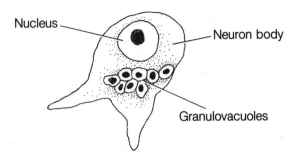

Nucleus

Neuron body

Granulovacuoles

Figure 5.   Granulovacuolar Degeneration in a Neuron.   Note that numerous granulovacuoles have formed in the body of this neuron around the nucleus.

cause a swelling of the cell's cytoplasm which may eventually lead to degeneration or dysfunction of the brain cell itself.

GVD and normal aging

With normal aging, GVD also appears in the hippocampal area, but its concentration and severity are relatively low, and this degeneration occurs at a relatively slow rate with aging (Kemper 1984). The rate of GVD is more rapid in Alzheimer's disease. Neurofibrillary tangles are also prevalent in the hippocampal area where high concentrations of GVD are found in Alzheimer's disease.

GVD and memory impairment. Occurs in diminished hippocampal cells

The severity of impaired memory functions associated with the hippocampus in Alzheimer's disease can be more fully appreciated when one considers that GVD occurs within an already shrinking population of neurons. More than one-half of the original neurons of the hippocampus may have been lost, which is suspected to be up to five times more serious than cell loss in normal aging (Ball 1983). Both GVD and tangles occur in this diminished cell population.

Role of hippocampus

The hippocampus is commonly given a major role in memory functions. Cells in the rear portion of the hippocampus, an area thought to be more involved in remote memories, are especially vulnerable to GVD. It thus appears that GVD may contribute to the disruption of more remote memories, a type of memory impairment that is most evident in later stages of Alzheimer's disease.

Future research and GVD

Though much remains to be discovered about GVD, some researchers believe it may have an even stronger relationship with certain types of behavioral deterioration than plaques and tangles (Ball 1983). This contention requires more investigation. Because GVD and tangles are closely matched in respect to their occurrence and location in the hippocampus, the possibility of related causes for both has been considered (Reisberg 1983). GVD was first described as a characteristic of dementia in 1911, but investigation of this abnormality in Alzheimer's disease is relatively recent. For that reason it has not received the attention given to the classic brain abnormalities of Alzheimer's disease, the tangles and plaques.

Hirano Bodies

Description of Hirano bodies

A fourth abnormality of Alzheimer's disease, first described by Hirano in 1965, is known as the Hirano body. This is a discreet type of change primarily seen in the hippocampus. A microscopic spindle-shaped structure (Kemper 1984), a Hirano body resembles a string of red blood cells (Davies and Wolozin 1987). Under an electron microscope, Hirano bodies appear to have a crystalline structure (Brun 1983). Hirano bodies invade the cell body of a neuron and also its processes (axons and dendrites). Neither the nature nor the importance of Hirano bodies has been clearly established although these abnormal structures have been associated with actin (Davies and Wolozin 1987), a major protein found in muscle fibers.

Age-related change

As with other abnormalities typical of Alzheimer's disease, the appearance of Hirano bodies in the brain is an age-related change. The bodies begin to appear in very small numbers during a person's teens, with a significant increase occurring only during and after the 60s. All persons over age 80 have Hirano bodies (Kemper 1984).

Hirano bodies and memory loss

Exactly how Hirano bodies affect the memory functions of the hippocampus is not known. However, some research suggests that Hirano bodies may trap ribosomes, rendering them dormant. Ribosomes are the agents that change RNA molecules—a basic unit of memory—into proteins, allowing the RNA to do its job of forming memories. If Hirano bodies are imprisoning the necessary ribosomes, then they may be preventing RNA from doing its job so that memories are not being formed. Further study testing this theory still is needed.

Congophilic Angiopathy

In this condition, amyloid is found deposited in cerebral blood vessels.

Amyloid, the problematic protein found in senile plaques, also appears deposited abnormally in the walls of cerebral arteries, capillaries, and tiny veins. Because amyloid is a congophilic material (one that picks up a dye known as congo red, used to identify tissues), the presence of these abnormal deposits in blood vessels is called congophilic angiopathy, or simply amyloid angiopathy (angiopathy meaning a disorder of the blood vessels).

Somehow related to Alzheimer's

The significance of congophilic angiopathy has not been clearly established, but there does appear to be some special connection between the deposits and Alzheimer's: while the condition appears in only 9 percent of neurologically normal individuals, it shows up in 92 percent of Alzheimer's patients. It also appears in all victims of Down's syndrome.

Angiopathy and strokes in Alzheimer's disease

We further know that congophilic angiopathy sometimes leads to hemorrhaging and infarction—tissue death caused by the obstruction of blood vessels—in the Alzheimer's brain. Infarction and hemorrhaging in turn can cause strokes, and strokes can result in dementia. Indeed, multi-infarct dementia—a condition resulting from multiple large or small strokes—accounts for about 15 percent of all dementing brain disorders (Reisberg 1981). A combination of multi-infarct dementia and Alzheimer's disease account for some 25 percent of all dementias in later life. Some researchers thus suspect that congophilic angiopathy is a contributing factor to stroke-induced dementia in Alzheimer's disease.

Possible causes of angiopathy

Other researchers theorize that congophilic angiopathy may signal an abnormality of the immune system of the brain or a deterioration of the blood-brain barrier, the special membrane that protects the brain from foreign substances. The deterioration of this barrier could cause both the angiopathy and the greater occurrence of infarcts and hemorrhage found in the Alzheimer's brain due to formation of amyloid deposits in the brain.

Major points

Research has identified five physical abnormalities of the brain—neurofibrillary tangles, senile or neuritic plaques, granulovacuolar degeneration, Hirano bodies, and congophilic angiopathy—that are consistently present in the brains of Alzheimer's patients. All are present in those parts of the brain that control memory and behavior, particularly in the hippocampus. Some of these same abnormalities also are found in other neurological illnesses that cause dementia and in Down's syndrome, which causes mental retardation. The eventual appearance of all of these abnormalities in the brain is an age-related change, and normal aging brains generally show similar changes although in much lower quantities.

No definite facts are known about the link between these observed abnormalities and the cause of Alzheimer's disease. However, because these abnormalities tend to occur in those areas of the brain that control the functions most affected by the disease, and because they might somehow destroy or disable brain cells, researchers believe they may explain much of the mental impairment suffered by Alzheimer's patients. If the breakdown of nerve cells in Alzheimer's disease can be better understood, it might be possible to prevent the degree of cell destruction in this disease. The chemical treatments currently under investigation depend to a large degree on functional nerve cells which decrease as the disease progresses. Research must still determine if the physical abnormalities represent the debris of this disease process, or if they contribute in some way to the destruction of what had been a functional mind.

Chemical Changes in the Brain

Accompanying the physical abnormalities that appear in the Alzheimer's brain are chemical changes: lowered levels of crucial chemicals that the brain requires to record, process, and store information. These chemicals have been found most significantly lowered in the areas of the brain most affected by Alzheimer's, leading researchers to strongly suspect that chemical changes cause some of the disease's impairments.

More about Brain Anatomy

Neurons send messages to and from the various areas of the brain.

At the cellular level, the brain is an intricate network of several billion interconnected cells, each equipped to perform a special task. Others included in this network are the billion or so nerve cells called neurons—the building blocks of a complex communication system that relays messages between the various areas of the brain and between the brain and the rest of the body. These messages travel along neuronal pathways. When plenty of healthy neurons are available to form the pathways, the whole communication system—and thus our thought processses themselves and other brain related abilities—can function properly. However, when large numbers of neurons deteriorate

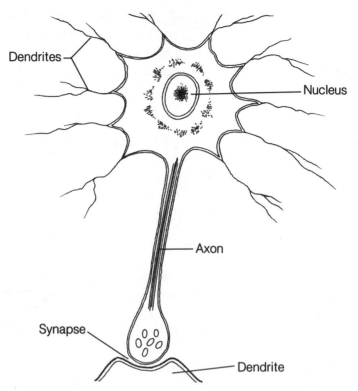

Figure 6. Example of a Neuron from the Brain. Note the axon, which carries the message a neuron sends to the synapse. Neurons have dendrites which receive message from other neurons. (The synapse where the axon and dendrite communicate with a neurotransmitter is enlarged so that the reader can visualize this area.)

or are destroyed, significant disruption of brain function occurs, severely limiting one's ability to think, act, and remember.

Neurons described   Neurons consist of a cell body and nucleus and protrusions called processes which transmit electrochemical messages from one cell to another. One kind of process, called an axon, sends a communication; the other called dendrites receive communications from other neurons (see Figure 6). Each neuron usually has a number

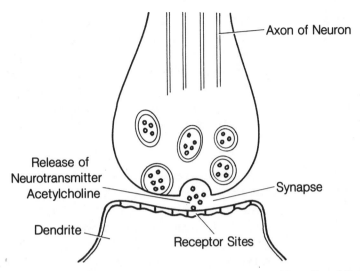

Figure 7.   A Neuron's Axon Shown Communicating with a Dendrite of Another Neuron.   Neurotransmitter is released into the synapse and picked up at dendrite's receptor sites. The neurotransmitter is made when the enzyme CAT (choline acetyltransferase) combines with acetyl to make acetylcholine, the neurotransmitter of the cholinergic system.

of dendrites (meaning tree with its branches). A remarkable feature of the brain's neurons is the fact that the axons and dendrites link neurons together in circuits. One neuron could conceivably transmit messages to literally hundreds of other neurons. Usually neurons are linked with only a few other recipient neurons. The body of the cell may also have connections with adjoining neurons and receive that neuron's message.

Synapse of a neuron   The actual transmission from an axon to the receiving part of another cell (dendrites or cell body) takes place in the tiny gap between them, called a synapse (see Figure 7). Neurons do not communicate directly by touching each other; the synapse is important because of what happens there. For a message to be conveyed in the special gap (synapse), a chemical message must be transmitted.

Neurotrans-
mitter

There is a specialized area at the end of a neuron's axon that secretes a chemical which combines with another chemical in that area of the synapse. The chemical process that occurs makes the neuron's special chemical messenger, a neurotransmitter. Without the neurotransmitter neurons could not communicate; the information these chemical messengers carry would not be conveyed.

Neurons in
pathways
using same
neurotrans-
mitters

Many neurotransmitters exist in the brain. Different neurons in the brain's network use different neurotransmitters. Neurons utilizing the same neurotransmitter form pathways in the brain, often arising from areas deeper in the brain that serve as a source of stimulation for a pathway of neurons using a common neurotransmitter to send messages. The neurotransmitter system thought to be involved in thought and memory is called the cholinergic system.

Alzheimer's
disease dis-
ables certain
neurons and
neurotrans-
mitters caus-
ing disruption
of the brain's
communication
system.

In Alzheimer's disease, problems develop in the brain's communication system. Disturbances or deficiencies in either the structural mechanisms (the neurons themselves) or the chemical messengers (the neurotransmitters) can lead to disturbances in behavior, thought, or emotion. In particular, Alzheimer's disables the brain's cholinergic system, which includes the neurotransmitter acetylcholine and its related network of neurons, known as the cholinergic neurons (Reisberg 1981) or the cholinergic system.

To a lesser degree the disease may also seem to affect the serotonergic system, which secretes the neurotransmitter serotonin; the noradrenergic system, which secretes the neurotransmitter noradrenaline (norephinephrine); and the system using the neurotransmitter somatostatin, which is also identified as a neuropeptide. In this section of the chapter, we will look at the changes wrought by Alzheimer's disease in each of these important chemical systems and at the subsequent disturbances in mental function and behavior that these changes appear to cause.

The Cholinergic System

Cholinergic neurons use the neurotransmitter acetylcholine. From a small area called the nucleus basalis of Meynert, these neurons and their processes reach up and out into the cortex of the brain. When these cholinergic pathways are not functioning, critical messages from one area of the brain to another cannot get through. Thus a healthy cholinergic system—the neurons and their associated chemical messengers—may be essential to our memory, thoughts, judgment, personality, sensory perception, and other higher mental functions. Certainly it is involved in memory and in giving information meaning.

Cholinergic neurons require the neurotransmitter acetylcholine and two enzymes—CAT and AChE—to communicate properly.

Cholinergic neurons communicate by means of a chemical chain reaction, and for the communication to work properly, all of the links in the chain must be in place. To start the process of transmitting information, a neuron secretes in its axon a chemical called acetyl (see Figure 8). The acetyl combines chemically with an enzyme known as choline acetyltransferase (CAT), and the CAT in turn creates the neurotransmitter, acetylcholine, which is released into the synapse. Acetylcholine, carrying its chemical message, is recognized by

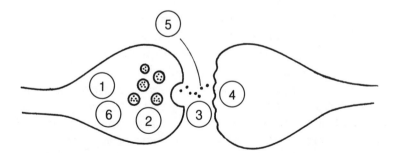

Figure 8. Neurotransmission. (1) CAT combines with acetyl, (2) Acetylcholine results, (3) Neurotransmitter released into synapse, (4) Receptors on receiving neuron picks up acetylcholine, (5) Enzyme AchE breaks down acetylcholine, (6) new transmissions begin the process again.

special sites (receptor sites) on the adjoining neuron. The message continues to be transmitted until another enzyme is activated. This enzyme is called acetylcholinesterase (AChE). Without the action of AChE on the acetylcholine, the neuron would be locked in to a message. Other messages could not be sent. Once the message is received by the adjoining cell and the acetylcholine is broken down, the whole process can begin again. It is this simple chemical system that enables the brain's network of neurons to send hundreds of messages throughout the body each minute.

In Alzheimer's disease these vital chemicals are lacking, leading to the destruction of cholinergic neurons.

In Alzheimer's disease, however, this system breaks down. For unknown reasons, the cholinergic neurons begin to lose both their acetylcholine neurotransmitters and the two vital enzymes, CAT and AChE. Research has shown that the cholinergic system in particular is attacked by Alzheimer's disease, and cholinergic neurons are selectively destroyed; however, the cause for this destruction remains puzzling. Also in question is the precise role that the breakdown of this system plays in causing the impairments associated with Alzheimer's disease.

Loss of CAT and AChE associated with impairment

Some research has focused on the loss of the enzymes CAT and AChE, finding that deficiencies of these enzymes tend to accompany physical abnormalities such as plaques and tangles. Cholinergic dysfunction in the hippocampus and in the frontal/parietal areas of the cortex is quite pronounced. Such deficiencies also have been found to correlate with Alzheimer's patients' degree of cognitive impairment and severity of dementia. This suggests that a reduction in enzyme activity alone may impair the cognitive and memory abilities of the whole cholinergic system.

Deficiencies in the enzymes CAT and AChE mean that acetylcholine can neither be made adequately nor effectively broken down again. The cholinergic system's functioning depends heavily on these enzymes carrying out their role effectively.

Origin of cholinergic system and impact of Alzheimer's

Scientists consistently agree that there is a tremendous loss of neurons using acetylcholine in Alzheimer's disease. Now we know that the origin of this system, the nucleus basalis of Meynert, suffers a loss of from 44 to 75 percent of its neurons. This area of the brain is the major source of cholinergic stimulation (Davies and Wolozin 1987; Tagliavini and Pilleri 1983; Coyle et al. 1983). A network of axons from neurons in the nucleus basalis forms cholinergic pathways up to the cortex. The substantial loss of neurons in the origin of cholinergic stimulation will reduce the stimulation to the cortex and hippocampus. Researchers cannot explain why neurons in close proximity to this special nucleus, which do not depend upon acetylcholine, show no significant damage.

When the amount of acetylcholine in the brain is low, patients lose their involvement with life.

Other research has concentrated on the neurotransmitter acetylcholine. This chemical appears to play a unique role in our ability to perceive our environment in a detailed and meaningful way (Restak 1984). It is connected with our ability to become intensely involved in the events around us and to remember what we experience—the appearance of a beautiful garden, perhaps, or the face of a new acquaintance. Conversely, when the amount of acetylcholine diminishes, Alzheimer's patients begin to lose their involvement with and enthusiasm for life. They become detached from the present and drift gradually into the past.

When cholinergic neurons are destroyed, patients suffer memory loss and other cognitive and emotional problems.

Unfortunately, deficiencies in one or more of these associated chemicals may lead to the destruction of the cholinergic neurons themselves. Once large numbers of neurons are damaged, the crucial neuronal pathways leading to and from the frontal/parietal and temporal lobes, the hippocampus, and other brain areas begin to shut down. Damage to the cholinergic pathways in and out of the hippocampus is particularly severe, leaving the hippocampus so isolated from the remainder of the brain that it might as well have been entirely removed (Hyman et al. 1984). This isolation most likely causes severe damage not only to memory functions but also to the patient's emotional health. It also may destroy necessary inhibitions, such as the fear of fire, that were learned through past emotional experience. In sum, damage to the cholinergic pathways linking the hippocampus with the cortex and the limbic structures, including the amygdala, as well as damage to other brain areas, seems to be responsible for much of the emotional and cognitive difficulty experienced by Alzheimer's patients.

The Serotonergic System

A loss of the neurotransmitter serotonin may cause sleep disturbances and mood changes.

Believed to regulate both sleep and sensory perception, the serotonergic system also shows disturbance in Alzheimer's disease. This system relies upon the neurotransmitter serotonin, which is also the chemical thought to induce sleep in the brain. Just as acetylcholine is deficient in the cholinergic system, serotonin has been found significantly reduced in a variety of brain areas when Alzheimer's disease is present (Volicer et al. 1985; Carlsson 1983). Also deficient is serotonin's metabolite (5-HIAA), which is a product of chemical changes related to metabolism. Some research suggests that deficiencies of these two chemicals are related to the sleep disturbances, mood changes, and overly aggressive behavior typical of some Alzheimer's patients (Volicer et al. 1985).

Link with Alzheimer's uncertain

The link between this system and Alzheimer's disease has not yet been as firmly established as the link with the cholinergic system. Current evidence, however, suggests that further research may well uncover important connections between deficiencies in the serotonergic system and Alzheimer's behaviors. For example, some researchers believe that persons with early onsets of dementia may be more likely to have deficiencies in other neurotransmitter systems in addition to the cholinergic system (Mohs et al. 1985).

The Noradrenergic System

Changes in Alzheimer's disease This system appears to counter the serotonergic system by triggering wakefulness and arousal. Too much of the operative neurotransmitter, noradrenaline, may produce severe stress reactions; too little may cause depression and excessive sleeping. One study reports that noradrenaline is reduced in the Alzheimer's brain by 57 to 74 percent (Gottfries 1985); another indicates that about half of all Alzheimer's patients suffer deficits of noradrenaline in the cortex, with a severe loss in only about 20 percent of that group (Davies and Wolozin 1987). The hippocampus and the hypothalamus also show deficiencies of noradrenaline, of from 49 to 73 percent (Winblad et al. 1982).

A lack of the neurotransmitter noradrenaline may cause emotional and sleep disturbances. Given the interplay of this system and the serotonergic system, disturbances in either or both neurotransmitters could cause the sleep disturbances found in Alzheimer's disease. Deficits of these chemicals could also explain why some patients become unusually heavily sedated by tranquilizers. On the other hand, a deficit of noradrenaline could also trigger emotional arousal. As with the serotonergic system, further research is needed before a definite link with Alzheimer's behaviors can be firmly established.

Somatostatin

Role in the brain and Alzheimer's disease Among the other neurotransmitter chemicals suspected of playing a role in Alzheimer's are the neuropeptides: somatostatin, substance P, neurotensin, and cholecystokin (Perry and Perry

1985). Neuropeptides are peptides made from amino acids which are now known to function as neurotransmitters in the brain.

A lack of somatostatin also appears to contribute to Alzheimer's dementia. In particular, a lack of somatostatin appears to accompany the disease and contribute some to its impairments. Although research on this chemical is still in the early stages, somatostatin has been shown to be significantly reduced in several brain areas, including the parietal lobe, a region thought by many to be affected first and most profoundly in Alzheimer's disease (Tamminga et al. 1987). Other recent findings suggest that a loss of somatostatin neurons may be directly related to Alzheimer's dementia (Tamminga et al. 1987). While many questions remain about the role of somatostatin, the most current research suggests that it may be second only to acetylcholine in its importance for Alzheimer's disease.

Treating Neurotransmitter Deficiencies

Drug interventions Some drug treatments already exist for treating deficits in the cholinergic system, although to date they have not proven particularly effective. It may be that this system needs to be treated in conjunction with other affected systems. As research into the disease and its effects on the brain continue, it is highly likely that other neurotransmitters and chemical systems that have a bearing on Alzheimer's disease will be discovered as well. Because the disease's symptoms can vary widely from one individual to the next, it may be that a number of different neurochemical deficiencies are involved. A given individual's symptoms could hold the clue to treatment: a patient suffering from early dementia, pronounced visual-spatial deficits, and lesser intellectual and memory impairment, for example, might be more responsive to cholinergic drug treatment alone.

Other drug treatments for other chemical systems are likely to be discovered.

As we learn more about the full range of neurotransmitter and other chemical deficiencies associated with Alzheimer's disease, it seems likely that drug treatments will become available which can at least partially compensate for these deficits and the problems they cause.

Summary

The levels of certain neurotransmitters and related chemicals crucial to the brain's information-communication process are lowered by Alzheimer's disease. The absence of these chemicals may cause the destruction of neurons, particularly the cholinergic neurons, that form the pathways to the hippocampus, the frontal/parietal lobes, and other areas of the brain's cortex. By cutting off effective communication between these areas, chemical disturbances in the brain may be responsible for many of the emotional, cognitive, memory, and behavioral changes suffered by Alzheimer's disease patients. Most Alzheimer's disease treatment-oriented research has sought ways to correct chemical abnormalities.

12

TREATMENT POSSIBILITIES

Role of drugs in Alzheimer's treatment
As medical researchers gradually come to understand the physical and chemical changes that occur in the Alzheimer's brain, they can use their knowledge to develop treatments that effectively prevent or reverse these changes. Many experimental studies using drug therapies on Alzheimer's patients already have been tried, with varying degrees of success. While no "wonder drug" for Alzheimer's disease—or even a clear and consistent treatment approach—has yet emerged, research has shown that some drugs help some of the people some of the time. Unfortunately, the studies completed thus far often show puzzling inconsistencies in response from one patient to the next. To achieve more consistent results, we no doubt need to learn more about the nature of the illness and its causes.

Cholinergic deficits target of treatment
To date, several major groups of drugs have been investigated. Many of the drug interactions in research have attempted to correct the deficiencies in the brain's cholinergic system. Since the neurotransmitter acetylcholine is deficient in the Alzheimer's brain and these deficiencies have been associated with Alzheimer's related impairments, it has been thought that finding ways to increase this chemical messenger might hold promise in treating the disease.

Basis for drug research   Additionally, lecithin and choline, which increase the availability of acetylcholine, have received some research attention. Drugs such as physostigmine and THA, which make acetylcholine available longer in the brain by blocking its destruction, have seemed promising in developing an effective treatment of Alzheimer's disease. Both drugs which directly increase the amount of acetylcholine and those that prevent its chemical destruction are called cholinergic agents.

Another type of drug treatment which is under study involves the manipulation of the cholinergic system. Drugs, called cholinergic receptor agonists, stimulate the receptors of a group of neurons which are specialized to communicate with the cholinergic neurotransmitter acetylcholine, thus enhancing its potency.

Much of the drug research in Alzheimer's disease has focused on the cholinergic system of the brain. Drugs (such as Naloxone) which affect other neurological systems have also been explored, but they have not delivered anticipated improvements. Additionally, other major groups of drugs, including vasodilators, neuropeptides, and psychostimulants, have been studied as to their positive effects on Alzheimer's patients.

In this chapter, we will look in turn at each of these groups of drugs and their effects. In addition, we will look at drug combination treatments and examine a nondrug therapy—neuronal transplants—that may hold a promise for the future. We also will discuss possible explanations for the inconsistent results of drug studies to date, including the possibility that Alzheimer's disease has distinct subtypes that respond to different treatments. First, however, we will discuss the issues that should be considered before one decides to participate in drug-research study.

Should You Participate in Drug-Research Study?

Participants in a drug-research study should carefully consider the risks and costs involved, as well as their own motivations.

In order for Alzheimer's treatments to be adequately developed and tested, it is necessary to conduct research using human subjects who have Alzheimer's disease. Subjects who volunteer for such studies do a great service both for medical research and for their fellow Alzheimer's sufferers. However, it is important that persons who elect to participate in a research study clearly understand the study's potential risks, results, and requirements, as well as their personal motivation for participating.

Families and subjects must not hold unrealistic expectations of significant improvement. Generally, persons with severe impairment have little chance of benefitting from drug treatment, while those in earlier stages of the disease may experience substantial, little, or no improvement. The drugs used might even cause a worsening of the patient's condition. Also, families and subjects sometimes cannot be told whether the subject will in fact be receiving the treatment medication or a placebo used for the control group.

Issues to consider

Other issues that must be carefully considered include:

- Purpose and rationale of study
- How study will be conducted
- Size and safety of dosage given
- Method of administering drug
- Potential side effects
- Responsibilities of the family
- Consent of the subject
- All expenses connected with participation (including travel, lodging, etc.)
- Researchers' attitude toward study participants (including family members)
- Researchers' credentials.

Inconsistencies in Drug Studies

Many unknown or uncontrolled variables may affect the results of studies, producing inconsistent findings.

Many uncontrolled variables exist in drug studies that may account for the frustrating inconsistencies found in Alzheimer's research. Among the many individual factors which may vary from one subject to the next, affecting or masking a drug's effects in a study include:

- Degree of subject's dementia
- Severity of loss of cholinergic neurons
- Incorrect diagnosis of Alzheimer's
- Coexisting disabilities (i.e., stroke)
- Other coexisting conditions (i.e., infection)
- Unrelated fluctuations in behavior and mood
- Age at onset of dementia.

Researchers do not yet know which variables may prove to be significant.

For example, a severe presenile dementia (onset before age 65) may be intrinsically different in terms of brain pathology than a severe senile dementia (onset after age 65), and thus it may respond very differently to a certain drug treatment. Any of the variables listed above may or may not prove to be an important indicator for Alzheimer's and drug research.

Other variables that must be controlled related to the study itself. These include:

- Dosage amounts
- Length of treatment and study
- Method of administration (oral, intravenous, etc.)
- Ways of measuring improvement
- Assumptions about the drug and effects expected
- Choice of symptoms to be measured.

Alzheimer's disease may prove to have distinct subtypes that respond differently to treatment.

Another possible explanation for the inconsistencies found is that Alzheimer's disease may have distinct subtypes, each associated with slightly different manifestations of symptoms and rate of progression. Different subtypes may respond differently to the same drug treatment. One researcher posits that two subtypes of Alzheimer's disease exist: AD-1 and AD-2 (Bondareff 1983). As defined, AD-1 begins in old age and follows a slow, subtle progression; AD-2 begins in middle age and shows a more rapid course and greater impairment. Other neurochemical and anatomical differences established between the two groups would seem to support this distinction. For example, AD-2 might develop under more genetically controlled influence.

Another researcher has suggested four distinct subtypes of the disease: extrapyramidal, myclonic, benign, and typical (Mayeux et al. 1985). As compared to the typical group, the extrapyramidal and myclonic groups each show certain accentuated features, while the benign group shows underexpressed features. The groups also differ as to severity of impairment in cognitive and memory functions.

Attention to subtypes may produce better treatment strategies.

Other researchers now are looking into the validity and significance of the subtypes, and overall, the concept of subtypes may prove rewarding to research treatments. It may be that attention to these subtypes, and to other distinguishing indicators such as age of onset and severity of dementia, will lead to the creation of better drug-treatment strategies with more predictable and reliable results.

Despite the many variables to be controlled and the inconsistencies found in studies to date, it has been shown definitively that drug therapies can produce improvements in Alzheimer's symptoms. The challenge now is to identify some clear pattern that will show us which drugs can be expected to help which patients, in what ways, and for how long.

Cholinergic Agents

As we saw in the Chapter 11 discussion of chemical changes, Alzheimer's disease is accompanied by a lowered level of the neurotransmitter acetylcholine in the brain. Insufficient acetylcholine causes dysfunction of the brain's cholinergic system, which may lead in turn to impairment of memory and cognitive abilities.

Cholinergic agents are drugs that increase the brain's level of acetylcholine.

Among the first treatments for Alzheimer's to be explored, then, are drugs that can increase the level of acetylcholine in the brain. The drugs tried include two substances that are precursors of acetylcholine: choline and lecithin. These substances increase the availability of acetylcholine. We will consider also physostigmine and THA which prevent the breakdown of this neurotransmitter. In this role, these two drugs prolong the availability of the acetylcholine. Finally, we will consider drugs that make the receptors for acetylcholine more sensitive, essentially heightening the potency of the available acetylcholine.

Choline

Choline therapy has produced extremely modest improvements.

A component of various foods and of commercially available lecithin, choline can increase the availability of acetylcholine in the brain and enhance its synthesis and release in synapses between the neurons. Because of these potential effects, it first was approached with a great deal of hope. In the numerous studies completed, however choline therapy has been associated only with extremely modest improvements in Alzheimer's patients or no improvements at all.

In some cases a modest increase in alertness and awareness has been reported, although the increase has been accompanied by mild irritability; in a few others, a reduction in confusion has been noted

(Fovall et al. 1983). But all of these improvements have been so mild that they could have been simply ordinary behavioral fluctuations unrelated to the choline therapy. Those patients who have appeared to improve were in the earlier stages of the illness; no effect from choline therapy seems possible in more advanced cases. Some research findings suggest that choline might prove more beneficial when used in combination with other drugs.

Side effects from choline include nausea, abdominal pain, diarrhea, incontinence, and fishy odor in the sweat. This last side effect has been avoided by substituting phosphatidylcholine, a more complex form of the drug of which choline is a component. The availability of choline and lecithin encourage their use.

Lecithin

Lecithin is a naturally occurring dietary substance found in many foods, including egg yolks, meat, fish, and soybean products. The dosages of lecithin used in treating Alzheimer's disease, however, are much higher than those obtainable through a healthy diet. Like choline, lecithin increases the availability of acetylcholine; it also raises the body's blood choline level and maintains that level longer than does straight choline (Etienne 1983). It has been shown to produce small improvements in some patients.

Lecithin appears to slow deterioration in some patients. The most important finding is that lecithin could be capable of slowing deterioration in a few patients. This may mean that long-term lecithin therapy can be used to slow down the disease's progress (Dysken 1987). Supporting this theory is the finding in the Dysken study that patients who discontinued use of lecithin showed more rapid deterioration. However, this very limited evidence must be replicated in other studies before stronger conclusions can be drawn.

Lecithin may be an effective supplement to other drug therapies. At present, lecithin treatment requires further exploration. No compelling evidence suggests that it alone can produce significant or consistent improvement, though it may prove an effective supplement to other drug therapies. (This will be discussed in a later section.) Furthermore, there is no scientific evidence in support of the idea that lecithin can prevent Alzheimer's. Lecithin therapy has shown some very modest improvements in some patients some of the time. The idea behind lecithin and choline, increasing the amount of acetylcholine, remains a promising direction for future research.

Side effects of lecithin can include nausea, diarrhea, irritability, and dry mouth. These are more likely to occur in older persons. Lecithin is not otherwise harmful. It can be purchased in health food stores, but that form is usually 20 percent lecithin (Henig 1981). It would be impossible to take enough of this form of lecithin to be of any benefit with Alzheimer's disease.

Physostigmine

How physostigmine works

This drug works by slowing down the chemical destruction of acetylcholine in the brain's synapses. By keeping the existing acetylcholine available longer, it increases cholinergic activity at active synapses, although it cannot help synapses that have been damaged or destroyed by the disease. Since physostigmine is thought to effectively cross the blood-brain barrier (Smith et al. 1979), it will be more effective in blocking the breakdown of acetylcholine by the enzyme, acetylcholinesterase.

Physostigmine has produced modest improvements in memory that are greater than the results with either choline or lecithin.

A danger of physostigmine is its narrow dose range: only a slight difference exists between a safe dose and one that is toxic. Additionally, it does not stay in the body very long; thus it must be given more frequently. Despite the disadvantages, more positive results have been achieved with physostigmine than with either choline or lecithin. The improvements noted are modest: in mid-sized dosed, it improves verbal recognition memory; in larger doses, it improves nonverbal recognition memory (Dysken 1987). Overall, it seems to have positive effects on visual memory, that is, memory of information that is presented in a visual form (e.g., recognizing pictures).

Physostigmine also seems to improve certain types of learning measured by psychological tests, and the improvement is the greatest in patients with only mild symptoms. It will not be as effective when other neurotransmitter systems are impaired in addition to the cholinergic system—a condition that seems to be more frequent with early onset dementia (Mohs et al. 1985).

Studies encouraging but variable Overall, the studies with physostigmine are encouraging. Because they have shown such widely varying kinds and degrees of improvement— including no improvement in many patients— further research is needed to pinpoint the best uses for this drug: the most effective doses, the types of functions improved by various doses, and the kinds of patients who respond best. It is now available to researchers in oral form. The potential for toxicity can be monitored although it remains a risk factor for physostigmine. Although this drug has not produced dramatic improvements and its effects on the progression of Alzheimer's disease have not been determined, physostigmine shows promise for further research.

THA

A recent THA study reports very positive results. THA (Tetrahydroaminoacridine) is perhaps the most exciting drug currently under study as an Alzheimer's treatment. A recent study reported fairly moderate improvement in many of the Alzheimer's subjects treated with this drug, and as these findings have been reported widely in the media, they have generated a great deal of interest and hope. It seems prudent, however, to approach THA with cautious optimism until the facts are more fully known.

How THA works THA has about the same chemical action as physostigmine: it slows the chemical destruction of acetylcholine in the brain's synapses. It has several advantages over physostigmine: (1) it is longer-acting (O'Conner 1986); (2) it has fewer side effects (Kaye et al. 1982; Sitaram et al. 1983); and (3) it also effectively crosses the blood-brain barrier (O'Conner 1986). THA can be taken orally. The fact that it can be taken orally (instead of by injection) and has few known side effects gives it a distinct advantage for use with the elderly population (Davis et al. 1982).

Early studies with THA alone did not all report positive results (Kaye et al. 1982). Improvement was more often reported when lecithin also was given; since lecithin increases the availability of acetylcholine and THA inhibits its breakdown, they may complement one another. However, larger doses of THA alone may be able to produce similar positive results (Rosenberg et al. 1983).

Sixteen out of 17 subjects treated with THA showed all-around improvement, and 10 showed moderate improvement.

In a 1981 study by Summers, 75 percent of the subjects (9 out of 12) showed subjectively measured improvement when treated with THA alone. In the most recent 1986 study of THA by Summers and his coworkers, 16 out of 17 subjects participating showed subjectively measured improvement. When the subjects were given objective psychological tests, 10 out of the 17 showed significant improvement, as compared with 7 out of 12 in 1981.

Too few studies have been done using THA; thus it is difficult to predict its effects on a larger population.

Despite the improvements reported in Summers' two studies, it is difficult to determine how effective THA may be in treating other persons with Alzheimer's. There just have not been enough research studies done using THA. A study by Kaye and others in 1982 indicated that less-impaired patients responded better. And in Summers' second study in 1986 the persons participating did not benefit equally. It appears that persons with more severe dementia did not respond as favorable as those with moderate dementia. The mean age of the subjects in the 1986 study was 71 years. Some of the subjects probably had an early onset (before age 65) of Alzheimer's disease. It is not known if these individuals benefited more or less from the THA treatment.

In Summers' 1986 study more subjects improved. Two reasons are given by Summers to explain this difference. First, better diagnostic techniques were used. Persons thought to have had Alzheimer's disease in the first study would have been excluded from the second study because they would not have met the criteria for an Alzheimer's diagnosis. Secondly, a more sensitive technique was used to determine the level of THA in the blood serum of subjects in the second study. This allowed Summers to better approximate a therapeutic level of THA.

Combination drug study with THA   One other point concerning the second THA study by Summers needs clarifying: THA was not the only drug given subjects in this study. Subjects were asked to take nine or more capsules of commercial lecithin (1200 mg per capsule) or its equivalent per day (Summers et al. 1986). Thus this THA study was actually a combination drug study. Lecithin would increase the availability of acetylcholine; THA would maintain its availability. The use of lecithin was based on one of its apparent components, phospholipids (O'Conner 1986). Phospholipids are essential for the construction of cell membranes to occur. Summers suggests that phospholipids may have a role in brain regeneration; even the Alzheimer's brain attempts to repair itself (O'Conner 1986).

Special actions of THA   THA may be different from physostigmine in several respects, which may enhance its ability to produce improvements in Alzheimer's patients. Because it may selectively block potassium channels in the central nervous system along with prolonging the life of acetylcholine, THA is suspected of playing a role in increasing the release of acetylcholine and prolonging the action potential of neurons releasing the neurotransmitter.

Side effects of THA and unknown effects   Side effects such as nausea, belching, abdominal discomfort, and diarrhea can occur with THA. These side effects can be eliminated by reducing the dosage and/or administering Robinul (Summers et al. 1986). The safety of THA and whether other side effects develop after long-term use have not been clearly established. Blood toxicity related to liver dysfunction and bone marrow suppression have been associated with this type of drug (*Lancet* editorial 1987). Although these potential side effects were not observed in Summers' studies, there is not yet sufficient long term use to rule out this possibility. THA studies involving more persons must be ready to contend with these side effects.

Inconsistencies with THA   No one yet knows whether a significant percentage of persons will show improvements by taking THA. Neither do we know whether the improvements reported in the last study by Summers can be sustained. Some patients in that study have experienced some deterioration even though therapy with oral THA continued. Since THA can only aid intact and active neurons, it seems likely that the gradual deterioration of neurons that accompanies Alzheimer's will eventually reverse the drug's effectiveness. Persons with greater loss of neurons may not respond favorably to THA. Most likely these individuals would have more advanced Alzheimer's disease with marked severity.

Still, THA appears to represent a positive direction for further research. We must learn more about its side effects. It may be possible to modify the drug's composition should significant side effects develop. Another very similar drug could be developed. In the meantime, we must consider mechanisms for more carefully controlled studies of THA.

Cholinergic Receptor Agonists

Studies of cholinergic receptor agonists have not produced significant improvements.   Other drugs that seem to help the brain's cholinergic system are cholinergic receptor agonists. These drugs work by stimulating the receptors that receive acetylcholine. Two such drugs, arecoline and RS-86, have been tried in studies on Alzheimer's patients, but unfortunately they produced little or no significant improvement (Bruno et al. 1986). Another drug, benthanechol chloride, did produce improvements such as decreased confusion, increased initiative, and greater productive activity in a four-subject study (Dysken 1987).

Administering drugs with a drug pump may allow more accurate research findings. One interesting aspect of the behthanechol study was the pioneering drug-administration technique used. A drug infusing pump was implanted into the subject's abdominal wall and connected to an intracranial catheter (Dysken 1987). The pump allowed the drug to reach the brain directly and to cross the blood-brain barrier; it also allowed direct measurement of the amount of drug in the brain, something impossible with other administration techniques. The pump's improved measurement abilities, together with the steady, guaranteed dosage it provides, may make it a more desirable administration technique for all studies of brain-altering chemicals, allowing more precise findings. These benefits, however, must be weighed against the undesirable physical intrusiveness of the pump and catheter.

Naxolone and Naltrexone

Naloxone and Naltrexone have not been shown effective against Alzheimer's. Treatment with these drugs represents a very sophisticated investigation of the role of more fundamental biological systems of the brain affected by dementing illnesses. Although they have been tried on Alzheimer's patients in several studies, they have failed to produce any real, consistent improvement. Only one study with Naloxone has shown significant benefits from the drug (Reisberg, Ferris, et al. 1983). Several others have found the drug to exacerbate undesirable symptoms. At present, there is little evidence to suggest that these drugs hold promise for future treatment.

Vasodilators and Nootropic Agents

Vasodilators improve blood flow to the brain. Vasodilators are a group of drugs that improves blood flow to the brain by expanding narrowed blood vessels. In a brain stricken by Alzheimer's disease, a rapid and diffuse reduction in cerebral blood flow occurs after the onset of symptoms; vasodilators can help offset this reduction. In fact, vasodilators are more effective in raising cerebral blood flow in Alzheimer's patients than in normal persons of the same age (Reisberg 1981) or in persons with arteriosclerotic brain changes often referred to as "hardening of the arteries."

Two types of vasodilators exist: primary and secondary. Primary vasodilators—such as Nylidrin, the only one drug shown to improve dementia—act directly on vascular deficiencies. Secondary vasodilators—such as hydergine and piracetam, discussed next—increase blood flow indirectly by stimulating cerebral metabolism. Metabolism is a chemical process necessary for the body and brain to maintain and regenerate themselves. Energy is a product of metabolism.

Cerebral blood flow has a strong relationship with metabolic activity. Disturbances in metabolism seem tied to reductions in cerebral blood flow found in Alzheimer's disease. For instance, persons with Alzheimer's have significantly lower levels of oxygen and glucose utilization in the frontal, temporal, and parietal areas of the brain. Secondary vasodilators stimulate the brain's metabolism to increase cerebral blood flow. The following secondary vasodilators show some promise for treating Alzheimer's disease.

Hydergine

Hydergine can improve the patient's mood, outlook, and possibly other symptoms. This is the drug most frequently prescribed for dementias of all kinds, and it is the medication most likely to be used with Alzheimer's disease by physicians. It has been studied extensively and shown to be extremely safe (Jenike 1985). Its effectiveness with dementias caused by strokes, however, has been questioned. Its major positive effect seems to be an antidepressant one. Significant improvements have been noted in many patients in such symptoms as emotional withdrawal, depressive mood, and motor retardation (Hutton 1987). Differing levels of improvements have been noted in a wider range of symptoms: mental alertness, orientation, anxiety, fear, motivation, initiative, agitation, vertigo, and locomotion. Occasionally, certain individuals show dramatic improvement (Jenike 1985); on the other hand, a few patients show a worsening of symptoms. Hydergine may seem to reverse the dementing process when actually it simply is improving the mood of the patients (and thus of those around them). Overall, response to this drug seems to vary greatly from one individual to the next.

Improvement generally is small. It generally takes several months before hydergine produces noticeable improvement, and even then the changes could be small rather than major. A six-month trial may be the most beneficial (Hollister and Yesavage 1984). If no clear benefits are seen after that time, use should be discontinued.

Piracetam

Another cerebral metabolic enhancer, piracetam is also one of the nootropic agents—a group of compounds that seems to improve functioning in mild to moderate senile dementia (Jenike 1985). Piracetam increases the response of neurons in the hippocampus (Cooper 1984) and appears to stimulate cerebral glucose metabolism (Jenike et al. 1986) and enhance release of acetylcholine in the hippocampus (Rosenberg et al. 1983).

Piracetam may improve memory and learning. In animal studies, piracetam has increased brain energy reserves, increased learning, and protected against learning impairment. The same studies indicate that piracetam does not have side effects or toxic effects at normal therapeutic doses (Schneck 1983). Preliminary evidence suggests that a combination of piracetam and choline given for one week improved memory storage, recall, and delayed recall (Schneck 1983). It may be that piracetam is most effective when combined with drugs that increase the availability of acetylcholine. As with other drug treatments, more mildly impaired patients—those whose cholinergic systems are least damaged and thus most responsive—seem to show the greatest benefit. This drug needs more research studies to determine whether it can be useful in treatment of Alzheimer's disease.

Neuropeptides

Neuropeptides are short chains of amino acids that have strong effects on the nervous system. Certain types of neuropeptides act as hormones in the body and have roles as neurotransmitters in the brain; they also assist in the communication between body cells, tissues, and organs (Reisberg 1981). Research into possible uses for neuropeptides in treating Alzheimer's is still in the early stages.

Neuropeptides may improve memory, learning, and mood, and hold promise as general geriatric antidepressants. In animal studies, neuropeptides have produced reversal of memory impairment. They also have been shown to boost human cognitive abilities, to play a role in neurotransmission, and in memory and learning. However, drug research with Alzheimer's patients to date has not had particularly encouraging results. Neuropeptides have been shown to produce mood improvements such as reduced depression, increased energy, and increased attention and concentration (Ferris 1983), and they may prove to have a role as geriatric antidepressants.

Vasopressin

Both a neuropeptide and a secondary vasodilator, vasopressin has improved memory and learning in animal studies. In one particularly interesting study with rats, vasopressin helped the animals remember things they had previously forgotten. In a study with Alzheimer's patients who suffered memory disturbances, use of a vasopressin nasal spray helped memories appear more quickly. Normal adult men have shown improved attention, concentration, and recall in response to vasopressin (Reisberg 1982).

Vasopressin and its analogs may improve memory, concentration, and mood. Vasopressin analogs—such as LVP, ODAVP, and DGAVP—also have been tried on Alzheimer's patients, with mixed results. One study has shown small but statistically significant improvements in memory, retrieval, and reaction time when an analog was administered (Ferris 1983). Possibly the more potent, longer-acting analogs will prove to have the greatest effects. Further research is needed to determine how vasopressin and its analogs work: by genuinely improving memory, by stimulating enhanced concentration, or by acting as an antidepressant.

Because of the role they seem to play in memory, learning, and communications between neurons, neuropeptides represent a promising frontier for further research. At the very least, they may prove helpful as antidepressant agents.

Psychostimulants

This group of drugs stimulated the central nervous system, increasing motor activity and reducing fatigue. Although psychostimulants do not improve cognitive or memory abilities, they can benefit other symptoms of Alzheimer's disease. Research has focused on treating three clusters of symptoms: (1) apathetic and withdrawn behavior, (2) mild depression, and (3) impaired short-term memory (Prien 1983).

Psychostimulants may improve attitude and mood. Of the psychostimulants tried, a number of drugs, such as ritalin, have generally proven unhelpful. These drugs may exacerbate behavior that is already agitated. Metrazol has received mixed reviews, but it has seemed to help with apathy, withdrawal, drive, and self-care (Prien 1983). However, it has a number of very undesirable side effects. Procaine hydrochloride, the primary active ingredient in a drug called Gerovital-H3, seems to have potential only for the treatment of geriatric depression (Prien 1983).

To date, then, psychostimulants have not proven particularly helpful, although they may have some use in treating specific subtypes of Alzheimer's. The side effects associated with these drugs require that they be carefully monitored, however, and may limit their usefulness.

Combination Drug Studies

Lecithin and THA seem to work well together, complementing each other's action. Often two or more drugs are given in combination so that each can help the other do its job. As we saw in the 1986 Summers study, for example, THA and lecithin were successfully combined to produce different but complementary actions. The lecithin increased the availability of acetylcholine in the synapses between neurons, while the THA inhibited the activity of the enzyme that breaks acetylcholine down in the receiving neuron. Together they produced the desired effect: more usable acetylcholine in the brain. In another study, lecithin and THA were given together to a group of Alzheimer's subjects with relatively high education and an average age of 61.5 years; some improvement in learning was noted, particularly among the more mildly impaired (Sitaram et al. 1983).

Lecithin has also been combined with choline and physostigmine. Lecithin has also been paired in studies with physostigmine. One study noted some improvements in long-term memory when lecithin and physostigmine were given together (Peters and Levin 1982). Another study of the same drug pairing produced even more impressive results. Eight out of the 12 subjects showed clear improvements in recall from long-term memory and a decrease in intrusions—memories seemingly forgotten but later interjected into another context (Thal and Fuld 1983). The results were repeated in a subsequent trial. Somewhat surprisingly, other studies of this drug combination have shown a greater degree of improvement in more severely impaired subjects.

Combination drug treatments, like single drug treatments, generally have not shown the kind of consistent results for which one might hope. Subjects who share similar characteristics—such as degree of dementia, early or late onset of dementia (before or after age 65), and so forth—do not seem to respond similarly to the drugs. This makes it very difficult to predict subject response or identify any pattern in the study results. Nonetheless, complementary drugs like lecithin and THA/physostigmine do seem to work better when paired than when used alone.

Neuronal Transplants

In the future, it may become possible to transplant healthy neurons to certain brain areas and thus regenerate brain function.

In the future, it may be possible to graft healthy neuronal tissue onto impaired areas of the Alzheimer's brain, thus stimulating the regeneration of neuron networks and improving certain brain functions. This transplant technique could offer an important alternative for more severely impaired victims, since drug therapies rarely seem to help those with extensive neuron damage.

Neuronal transplants already have been tried on subjects suffering from Parkinson's disease. One such study reported a slowing of degeneration (Moore 1987), while another reported an improvement in motor functioning (Madrazo et al. 1987). Animal research with neuronal transplants has shown that the technique can achieve desired results for specific behavioral and cognitive impairments (Gash et al. 1985; Merz 1987; Fine 1986; Gage et al. 1984).

Finding sources for donor tissue raises delicate ethical questions.

Before neuronal transplants can be widely used, however, the sensitive issue of donor tissue must be resolved. In the latest Parkinson's disease study, dopamine-producing cells were simply transplanted from the patient's own adrenal glands. An equivalent source of acetylcholine-producing cells from the patient's own body for treating Alzheimer's disease is not yet known if it does exist. It may be possible to use fetal brain tissue from some other animal; an even better source of donor tissue would be the brains of aborted human fetuses. Animal studies with grafted fetal tissue have been quite successful, although the technique has not been tested with human neuronal tissue. The use of either animal or fetal tissue, however, raises serious moral and ethical questions that would first have to be addressed.

Most likely, years of animal research will need to be completed before experimentation with human subjects can even be considered. Perhaps in that time, the ethical questions surrounding this treatment possibility will be answered as well. Neuronal transplants are an experimental possibility for research at this time.

13

PSYCHIATRIC MEDICATIONS AND DEMENTIA

Psychiatric medications can be effective in managing some symptoms of Alzheimer's. Psychiatric medications can be effective in managing some symptoms of Alzheimer's disease. An overview of these various medications will be helpful to caregivers. Since side effects, some quite adverse, can develop, these medications require close monitoring by physicians and family members. Individual responses to psychiatric medications can vary considerably, from clear benefits, to no change, to even worse symptoms. The elderly generally have a lower tolerance for these medications than younger persons, and brain impairments often interfere with the effectiveness of a medication.

A good rule of thumb with psychiatric medications is to start persons at low dosages, increasing dosages slowly. This approach may be frustrating to family members who are seeking rapid relief from some symptoms. It is a safer approach, however, and allows physicians to monitor an individual's response to a medication. Side effects are more likely to occur at higher dosages. If the person is going to experience adverse side effects, these probably will occur in a milder form at a lower dose. Additionally, it is critical to determine over a period of time whether a person can tolerate a specific psychiatric medication; lower doses allow the body to gradually adjust to the medication.

No one but a physician should change prescribed dosages. Only physicians should change dosages. Family members should consult the physician if side effects develop or if the medication is simply not working. Families should have realistic expectations about changes they can expect; generally medications can produce moderate changes. Target symptoms should be discussed with the prescribing physician, who must be informed of any other medications the patient is currently taking. Family must not change the dosage even if behaviors such as agitation or angry outbursts are still occurring. In fact, more of the medication could create more severe symptoms, which is especially true with major tranquilizers. Administering more medication than prescribed can also create more side effects, which can be dangerous, especially for the person with Alzheimer's disease. The following example illustrates some problems associated with increasing the dosage of a major tranquilizer without the advice of a physician.

A case example illustrating the harmful effect of too high a dosage of a major tranquilizer Emma Day, an elderly woman, had been prescribed a 150 mg total daily dosage of a major tranquilizer. This particular medication (Mellaril) had high sedative effects. The dosage had been increased over a month to reduce symptoms of agitation, sleeping difficulties, and delusional beliefs about her husband. These symptoms were reduced but still occurred occasionally. Jim, the husband, had diabetes and severe arthritis. The diabetes was not well-controlled, thus causing periods of depression.

On this particular day, Jim was somewhat agitated himself due to fatigue and worry over caregiving and financial problems. He was abrupt and aggravated with Emma's slowness in bathing. He saw her behavior as resistant and uncooperative. As he became more forceful, Emma became more upset. The more he pushed, the more hostile she became. Later she calmed down, but Jim decided on his own to increase her medication. That night he doubled the dosage.

The next morning Emma was a little more confused and sedated; Jim doubled the dosage again. Later that morning she was still in bed, and Jim wanted her to get up. He got her out of bed with some difficulty, pointed her toward the bathroom, and left for another part of the house. On his way he heard her fall. She was not seriously injured, but her shoulder and elbow were badly bruised. For several weeks, Jim had to help her more with dressing and bathing. Emma's fall and Jim's increased workload were direct results of too much tranquilizer given without a doctor's order.

Major tranquilizers generally should not be used as chemical restraint. Except in extraordinary circumstances the use of major tranquilizers as a chemical restraint is inappropriate. This should never be done at home by family members. Two other points are made in the example above: (1) caregivers, particularly those who are older, often have health problems that can interfere with caregiving and their response to daily stressors, and (2) it is to the benefit of the caregiver and patient to use problem-solving and coping skills, rather than to increase medication.

In this chapter, we will cover three groups of medications used in treating symptoms associated with dementia or other coexisting psychiatric conditions, such as depression. Side effects will be discussed and listed by groups of medications that may produce them. The reasons these medications are prescribed, as well as their generic and brand names, will be noted.

Side Effects

Major tranquilizers are the most frequently prescribed medications for symptoms associated with dementia. One potential side effect that must be monitored is *hypotension*. This results in a lowering of blood pressure, which can increase the risk of falls caused by dizziness and loss of balance.

Another type of side effect is called *extrapyramidal reactions,* which causes decreased or slowed movements, muscle rigidity, resting hand tremor, shuffling gait, drooling, and a mask-like face. Some of these symptoms can accompany dementia particularly if true Parkinson's disease coexists with Alzheimer's disease. The drug-induced or "pseudoparkinsonism" is likely to appear sometime between the first week and two months after beginning treatment with a major tranquilizer. These symptoms can be reduced with careful additions of other medications, which in turn may be discontinued later if the symptoms fade.

When major tranquilizers are given to reduce agitation and restlessness but instead produce these symptoms, the person is having a "paradoxical reaction" to the medication. The patient cannot sit still, may be constantly pacing, and feels anxious and agitated. In addition, the person may find it difficult to sleep; no position is comfortable. A change in medication, reducing the dosage, or use of an antiparkinson-type medication might help some people with this side effect.

If persons with Alzheimer's disease have taken major tranquilizers for a long time, they run the risk of another type of extrapyramidal reaction called "tardive dyskinesia." Advancing age can also be a risk factor. This type of side effect is characterized by involuntary lip and tongue motions and writhing movements of the arms and legs. In more severe tardive dyskinesia speech, eating, walking, and even breathing can be impaired. Reducing the dosage or adding an antiparkinson medication does not consistently help reduce this side effect. The best treatment is preventive; that is, avoid the use of major tranquilizers whenever possible or use low dosages.

Another possible side effect is a delirium or reversible dementia that is related to an anticholinergic effect some major tranquilizers can have. The more common features involve dry mouth, blurred vision, dilated pupils, constipation, urinary retention, nasal congestion, and increased heart rate. A few major tranquilizers can inhibit ejaculation. The cholinergic system of the brain, which is vital to memory functions, is already impaired in Alzheimer's disease. Major tranquilizers and some classes of antidepressants block the function of acetylcholine, the chemical messenger intrinsic to the cholinergic neurons of the brain.

In addition, a syndrome can develop which appears as an acute, toxic confusional state. This state is characterized by disorientation, visual hallucinations, irritability, and impaired attention. The syndrome can be treated by discontinuing the drug(s) with anticholinergic effects. Symptoms should clear in two to three days. The medication can then be changed to one with less anticholinergic properties or resumed if the syndrome developed from a toxic buildup.

Several other side effects can occur with some major tranquilizers. One which applies particularly to elderly persons is greater sensitivity to heat and cold. Weight gain can also occur when taking major tranquilizers. Cardiac side effects, while rare with some of the major tranquilizers, are possible and must be taken into consideration for those patients with heart conditions.

Other side effects can occur but are quite rare. Family members should consult a physician when the Alzheimer's patient is prescribed any type of medication in order to monitor side effects.

Three groups of psychiatric medications, major tranquilizers, minor tranquilizers, and antidepressants, are described in the tables that follow.

Major Tranquilizers
(Neuroleptics or Antipsychotics)

Purpose: Manage symptoms of agitation/anxiety, suspiciousness, hostility, delusions, hallucinations, preoccupations, poor self-care resulting from psychotic state, social withdrawal, uncooperativeness, belligerent and hostile behavior.

Drugs have a tranquilizing or sedating effect. There is an antipsychotic effect or normalizing effect on mood, thought, and behavior.

Side Effects:

Drowsiness	Sensitivity to light	Decreased sweating
Dry mouth	Shakiness	Difficulty urinating
Constipation	Muscle spasms in neck/back	Restlessness
Blurred vision	Dizziness/light-headedness	Hypotension
Stiffness	Stuffy nose	Fast heartbeat
Drooling	Decreased sexual ability	Shuffling gait

Any side effects of concern should be brought to the attention of the physician prescribing the medication. The following table notes some common major tranquilizers and side effects.

MAJOR TRANQUILIZERS

Trade Name	Generic Name	Sedative	Anticholinergic	Extrapyramidal
High Potency				
Haldol	Haloperidol	Low	Low	High
Navane	Thiothixene	Low	Low	High
Prolixin	Fluphenazine HCL	Low	Low	High
Stelazine	Trifluoperazine HCL	Moderate	Low	Moderate
Moderate Potency				
Trilafon	Perphenazine	Moderate	Moderate	Moderate
Loxitane	Loxapine Succinate	Moderate	Moderate	Moderate
Moban	Molindone HCL	Moderate	Moderate	Moderate
Low Potency				
Thorazine	Chlorpromazine	High	High	Low
Mellaril	Thioridazine	High	High	Low

Minor Tranquilizers

Minor tranquilizers are used to treat some symptoms that accompany Alzheimer's disease. They may be more appropriate for controlling anxiety/agitation when psychotic features are not evident. These medications can build up in the body over time, thus those medications with a shorter half-life should be used to prevent this buildup. The longer the half-life of a medication, the longer it stays in the body. We will note the half-life below and each drug's action rate (rate of onset). In some cases, it may be more appropriate to dispense this medication as needed rather than regularly. We will only note the antianxiety agents.

Purpose: Reduce symptoms of anxiety/agitation and related insomnia.

MINOR TRANQUILIZERS

Generic Name	Brand Name	Rate of Onset	Half-Life (Hours)	Dose Range mg/ day for Elderly
Diazepam	Valium	Fastest	26–53	2–10
Clorazepate dipotassium	Tranxene	Fast	30–200	7.5–15
Triazolam	Halcion	Fast	2–5	.25–.5
Lorazepam	Ativan	Intermediate	20–200	.5–4
Chordiazepoxide HCl	Librium	Intermediate	8–28	5–30
Alprazolam	Xanax	Intermediate	6–15	.125–.5
Oxazepam	Serax	Intermediate to slow	5–15	10–30
Temazepam	Restoril	Intermediate to slow	12–24	15–30
Prazepam	Centrax	Slow	30–300	10–15

Side Effects:

Oversedation	Dizziness	Fatigue
Drowsiness	Light-headedness	Depression
Unusual excitement	Headache	Blurred vision
Nervousness	Irritability (paradoxical)	Breathing problems

As with other medications, use of minor tranquilizers may not be appropriate with other medical conditions. The physician will consider this factor. Withdrawal from this type medication should be supervised by a physician since there can be problems if the person has taken the medication for a long time.

Antidepressants

While there is some question about how often Alzheimer's patients are depressed, there is no question that depression can precede or coexist with Alzheimer's disease. Some depression (coexisting with Alzheimer's disease) can be treated successfully, and the person's mental status will improve. However, side effects are a major

ANTIDEPRESSANTS

Generic Name	Brand Name	Sedation	Anticholinergic	Cardiovascular
Amitriptyline	Elavil	High	High	High
Doxepin	Sinnequan Adapin	High	High	Moderate
Nortriptyline	Aventyl/Pamelor	Moderate	Moderate	High
Imipramine	Tofranil	Moderate	Moderate	High
Desipramine	Norpramin	Low	Low	Moderate
Protriptyline	Vivactil	Very Low	Moderate	High
Maprotiline	Ludiomil	Moderate	Moderate	Moderate
Amoxapine	Asendin	Moderate	Moderate	Low
Trazodone	Desyrel	High	Very Low	Very Low

concern with antidepressants. Anticholinergic effects can occur with antidepressant medications. While all side effects can be significant, those that produce more confusion and delirium must be prevented. In dementia, these effects compound existing memory and cognitive deficits. Careful use of the appropriate antidepressants can sometimes avoid these side effects. (See Chapter 3 for more detailed information about depression with Alzheimer's.)

Purpose: Decrease aspects of depressed mood, improve appetite and sleeping habits, improve social functioning, increase level of energy.

Side Effects:

Drowsiness
Dry mouth
Urinary retention
Nasal congestion
Delirium
Increased appetite for sweets

Increase in heart rate
Blurred vision
Constipation
Dizziness/fainting
Tremors
Slow pulse

Hypotension
Arrythmias
Weight gain
Stomach upset
Nausea

There is some interest in another type of antidepressant medication, the monamine oxidase inhibitors (MAOs or MAOIs). This antidepressant may be considered when others do not work. However, special care must be taken regarding dietary restrictions and combining with other medications. This type of medication also has side effects which must be carefully considered.

Most antidepressant medications take several weeks to a month to reach a therapeutic level. Families must take this into account and be patient. With the elderly, a lower dosage is often initiated to determine how well the antidepressant will be tolerated.

Summary

Psychiatric medications—when carefully prescribed and monitored—can be helpful in the management of psychiatric symptoms associated with Alzheimer's disease. Family must understand why these medications are prescribed and what side effects can be expected. Many times a simple explanation will encourage Alzheimer's patients to take their medications. All psychiatric medications can help with "nerves," relaxation, and sleep. Families must be responsible for monitoring side effects and reporting these to the prescribing physician. Family members must avoid the temptation to exaggerate or overreport disturbing symptoms in order to increase prescribed dosages. Finally, the help of a professional should be sought to learn more appropriate ways to handle behavior problems and caregiver stress. Depending solely on psychiatric medications will not be sufficient.

APPENDIX A

WORKSHEETS

Use of the Behavior Profile

The "Behavior Profile" can be helpful to the family caregiver and professional. We will briefly discuss its contents and uses.

Behavioral areas: There are 58 behaviors listed in five categories. These behaviors occur with Alzheimer's disease although some may not occur as frequently in all persons. Certainly on an infrequent basis some occur with almost everyone. The difference is frequency. The behavior problem can occur with other conditions, particularly psychiatric disorders.

How often it occurs: Many problems are not significant unless they occur frequently. This is certainly the case with symptoms and their manifestations in Alzheimer's disease. More supervision may be indicated if a behavior occurs frequently, such as not eating or bathing; others need attention even if a behavior occurs infrequently, such as wandering or leaving the stove turned on. The caregiver can use the frequency of a behavior to plan the necessary degree of assistance and supervision. Some behaviors will require more intervention than others. Potential consequences of a behavior will influence the type of intervention and how quickly an intervention must be made. For instance, if a person begins to get lost driving, action must be taken to stop his driving. Denial of problems may occur. This will be bothersome but does not pose a problem unless the person insists on doing things anyway that could have harmful consequences.

How much it bothers you: This will help point out behaviors that need more understanding and attention. For instance, if toileting accidents are extremely bothersome to the caregiver, this area should be addressed to reduce the number of accidents. If the person has delusional ideas, these will probably be accompanied by agitation. These behaviors usually bother caregivers a great deal initially. Psychiatric medication will probably be needed. As caregivers are trying to adjust to the symptoms of Alzheimer's disease, they may be bothered more by a larger number of symptoms.

Completing the profile: For each behavior, check the most appropriate box under the two categories: *How often it occurs* and *How much it bothers you.* If the behavior is no longer a concern because you have taken over that area, scratch through the behavior and the row of boxes to the right. For example, if you pay bills for the person now, scratch through "forgets to pay bills" and the boxes to the right.

Use of the profile: Both caregivers and professionals can use the profile. Caregivers can complete the profile and refer to it to see how behaviors change and how their perception of problems change. The more seriously impaired person will have more behaviors occurring more frequently. This, however, usually occurs over time. If the frequency of numerous behaviors increases abruptly, an underlying medical condition may have developed. Medications might need to be reviewed.

If the person has not been diagnosed, the completed profile will provide information to the physician about the individual's functioning and the caregiver's concerns. The profile is not intended to be a diagnostic tool, but when a person is not testable, a reliable family informant can provide a more complete picture of functioning by completing the profile.

For counseling purposes the profile can indicate behaviors that need more problem-solving work and understanding. It also more quickly identifies behavior areas that are of great concern to the caregiver and thus require additional support and/or intervention.

BEHAVIOR PROFILE

NAME: _____ CAREGIVER: _____

DATE: _____ LENGTH OF CAREGIVING: _____

Check the appropriate category for each behavior.

BEHAVIORAL AREAS	How Often It Occurs				How Much It Bothers You				
	Always	Usually	Sometimes	Never	Extremely	Very much	Moderately	A little	Not at all
ORIENTATION									
1. Fails to recognize friends									
2. Fails to recognize family									
3. Forgets year									
4. Forgets month									
5. Forgets day of week									
6. Unable to name place (town, etc.)									
7. Fails to recognize familiar places									
8. Gets lost in neighborhood (walking)									
9. Gets lost driving									
10. Gets lost in own home									
11. More confused at night									
12. More confused in new places									
13. Wanders and gets lost									
MEMORY									
14. Loses/misplaces small items									
15. Loses/misplaces valuable things									
16. Forgets to pay bills									
17. Forgets to eat									
18. Unable to recall what was read									
19. Forgets to turn things off									
20. Forgets what conversation is about									
21. Unable to follow what's on TV									
22. Forgets to bathe									
23. Forgets major events of the day									
24. Forgets major events of the week									
25. Forgets major events from distant past									
LANGUAGE									
26. Unable to initiate conversation									
27. Misunderstands what others say									
28. Unable to respond to questions									
29. Has trouble finding right words									
30. Just speaks in phrases									
31. Avoids questions									

	How Often It Occurs				How Much It Bothers You				
	Always	Usually	Sometimes	Never	Extremely	Very much	Moderately	A little	Not at all
32. Unable to verbalize needs									
33. Repeatedly says same things									
34. What is said makes little sense									

AMBULATION/MOVEMENT

	Always	Usually	Sometimes	Never	Extremely	Very much	Moderately	A little	Not at all
35. Walks short, shuffling gait									
36. Gait slow and labored									
37. Tires easily when walking									
38. Unable to get up from chair alone									
39. Unable to use stairs									
40. Unable to use eating utensils									
41. Unable to write name									
42. Hands/arms shake									

BEHAVIOR PROBLEMS

	Always	Usually	Sometimes	Never	Extremely	Very much	Moderately	A little	Not at all
43. Has problems sleeping									
44. Has toileting accidents									
45. Talks excessively about past									
46. Denies problems									
47. Gets upset easily									
48. Becomes physically violent									
49. Shows poor judgment									
50. Has trouble taking medication									
51. Drives unsafely									
52. Very withdrawn, refuses to leave house									
53. Very nervous and restless									
54. Walks and paces constantly									
55. Very suspicious/paranoid									
56. Has delusional ideas									
57. Has hallucinations									
58. Sexually inappropriate									

OTHER

	Always	Usually	Sometimes	Never	Extremely	Very much	Moderately	A little	Not at all
59.									
60.									
61.									
62.									
63.									

Using the Personal/Social Support Resources

Family members often become isolated in caregiving; however, this is not inevitable. Contact with the outside world can be maintained. As stress and pressures of caregiving build, it is difficult to think of who can help. Thus it is a good idea to identify persons to call on for assistance before you become overwhelmed by too many demands and have no time to think.

First, it is helpful to evaluate the supports within the family and neighborhood. As independent people, many caregivers like to think they can always take care of themselves, but constant caregiving can change things. They may need much more support and help; That is when caregivers can turn to family, friends, neighbors, church members, or professionals for help.

We have found in our work that it is often difficult initially for caregivers to complete this form. Too often, only one person is the support for all areas covered by the questions. It is important for others to be considered as backup resources and for the caregiver to begin to rely on at least one or two people to cover some of the areas. Family support groups can be important resources.

Some of the questions point to a need for a more immediate source of security. For example, when the caregiver is frightened, he or she needs to talk to someone quickly. If the behavior of the relative is threatening, the caregiver may want to call the doctor or mental health professional. If the caregiver suspects a burglar is in the house, he or she must call the police.

Different resources may be more appropriate for different questions. Caregivers are encouraged to use this form to examine closely their total support network. A confidant is a valuable resource, but other personal resources may need to be developed.

PERSONAL/SOCIAL SUPPORT RESOURCES

NAME: _____ DATE: _____

Using your own situation, check the most appropriate Personal/Social Supports to the right of each question. Try to check at least 3.	Yourself	Spouse	Children	Other Family	Friends	Neighbors	Church	Pastor/Priest	Doctor	Other Professional	Support Group	Agency Staff	Other
1. Who can you count on for transportation?													
2. Who can you count on for financial help/decisions?													
3. Who helps most with household chores?													
4. Who can you count on to get to appointments?													
5. Who do you enjoy doing things with during the week?													
6. Who can you count on in time of crisis?													
7. Who can you count on when you're physically sick?													
8. Who can you count on to console you when you're very upset?													
9. Who would you seek out when you're frightened?													
10. Who would you talk to when you're lonely?													
11. When you need to talk, who can you count on to listen?													
12. With whom can you really be yourself?													
13. Who do you trust completely?													
14. Who do you feel really appreciates you as a person?													
15. With whom do you have the most frequent contact?													
16. Whose advice are you most likely to accept?													
17. Who supports your independence the most?													

Using your own situation, check the most appropriate Personal/ Social Supports to the right of each question. Try to check at least 3.	Yourself	Spouse	Children	Other Family	Friends	Neighbors	Church	Pastor/Priest	Doctor	Other Professional	Support Group	Agency Staff	Other
18. Who seems to understand you best?													
19. Who helps you to be honest with yourself?													
20. Who helps you keep a positive outlook?													
21. Who do you enjoy being with the most?													
22. Who best understands your current situation?													
23. Who helps you work out your problems most?													
24. Who could temporarily take your place in caregiving?													
25. Who do you trust regarding legal matters?													
26. Who can you talk to about family problems?													

In-Home Care List

This form may be used by family members to determine how much assistance their relatives actually need to perform activities of daily living. Realistic expectations can develop, and this information can be communicated to other persons who help with caregiving. Alzheimer's patients should be encouraged to do what they can for themselves; family members must avoid doing things for them unnecessarily.

Some persons with Alzheimer's disease still live alone. In these cases, the "In-Home Care List" will help family members to determine how much assistance the person needs.

Nursing homes can use this form to get a better idea of how much assistance the resident will require in daily living activities, socialization, and leisure/recreational activities. This scale is a planning, communication, and monitoring tool. Other professionals may use it to help families secure appropriate community resources.

For each behavior check the category that best describes how it occurs. For example, for the behavior to occur appropriately or as one desires, verbal assistance, physical assistance, or complete supervision may be necessary. On the other hand there may be no need for assistance of any kind for the behavior to occur as desired on a regular basis. In some cases the behavior may not be carried out as desired or appropriately even with complete supervision. In that case one should check that the behavior does not occur appropriately. Put NA for "not applicable" when that behavior does not apply.

Definitions

Without assistance: The behavior occurs appropriately with no assistance or corrective devices (e.g., glasses, hearing aid, walker, etc.).

With verbal assistance: The behavior occurs appropriately or as desired with *only* verbal cues, reminders, instructions, directions, and so forth.

With physical assistance: Verbal assistance is not enough; physical assistance is required for the behavior to occur appropriately; the caregiver physically assists or does for the person; glasses and other adaptive devices represent physical assistance.

With total supervision: The behavior occurs only if totally supervised. Both verbal and physical assistance may be necessary as part of the supervision.

Behavior does not occur appropriately: The behavior does not occur as desired even with assistance and supervision.

IN-HOME CARE LIST

NAME: _____   DATE: _____

| | Behavior Occurs Appropriately: | | | Behavior Does Not Occur Appropriately |
	Without Assistance	W/Verbal Assistance	W/Physical Assistance	W/Total Supervision	
I. Activities of Daily Living					
Basic					
A. Dresses self					
B. Bathes regularly					
C. Eats regular meals					
D. Takes prescribed medication					
E. Takes over-the-counter medications					
F. Uses bathroom as necessary					
G. Grooms self regularly					
H. Wears clean clothing					
Advanced					
A. Prepares meals					
B. Does food shopping					
C. Pays bills					
D. Uses telephone					
E. Uses stove safely					
F. Follows medical advice					
G. Handles money					
H. Washes clothes					
I. Keeps house clean					

J. Follows daily routines
K. Wears suitable clothing for weather
L. Seeks help when needed
M. Drives car
N. Has regular contact with doctor

II. Socialization
A. Leaves house for social activities
B. Good interaction with friends, neighbors
C. Good interaction with spouse
D. Good interaction with other family
E. Expresses self
F. Understands what others say
G. Recognizes familiar people
H. Generally gets along with people

III. Leisure Activities
A. Follows specific instructions
B. Walks in yard
C. Walks in neighborhood
D. Reads newspaper
E. Watches TV
F. Plays games
G. Looks at magazines
H. Enjoys gardening
I. Listens to music
J. Enjoys arts and crafts
K. Does exercise
OTHER:

Care Management Stress

This form can be useful for the family caregiver and professionals involved with the caregiver and the Alzheimer's patient. It is another approach to problem solving and making changes in the caregiver situation. Some changes must occur as a result of psychological adjustment, but family support and outside resources can help. For example, when it is hard to accept the diagnosis of Alzheimer's, the caregiver needs time to adjust and plenty of information in order to understand what lies ahead for both patient and caregiver. For a caregiver who experiences frequent financial problems, family meetings to discuss possibilities and an investigation of community resources may prove helpful.

When a caregiver often feels isolated and abandoned, other people showing their care and concern can help. Other statements reflect the caregiver's response to frequent stress. Another cluster of statements may suggest depression or other adjustment problems that may require professional treatment. For example, being overly upset or fatigued, sleeping poorly, or feeling nervous, all suggest the need for more support, counseling, and perhaps treatment for the caregiver.

Family problems or feelings of estrangement may be evident if statements concerning family are rated frequently. These kinds of problems may require counseling or other approaches to bring the family back together or to develop ways to accept dissenting family views.

This stress scale can assist caregivers in assessing how they are coping over the duration of the caregiving experience.

CARE MANAGEMENT STRESS

CAREGIVER: _____ DATE: _____ AGE: _____

CLIENT: _____ AGE: _____ DURATION OF CAREGIVING: _____

Please check a response for each.

	NEVER	RARELY	SOMETIMES	FREQUENTLY	NEARLY ALWAYS
1. I'm uncomfortable leaving my relative alone.					
2. Worries bother me a lot.					
3. I get tired and worn out doing everything.					
4. Family fail to understand what I'm experiencing.					
5. Everyone fails to appreciate what is happening.					
6. Family members could help a lot more.					
7. I'd like to see friends more.					
8. My relative's behavior frightens me.					
9. It's hard now to accept this diagnosis.					
10. It's hard for my family to accept this diagnosis.					
11. I'm feeling more tense and nervous.					
12. I have a lot of financial concerns.					
13. My relative asks too much of me.					
14. I feel abandoned by doctors/professionals.					
15. I feel my health is suffering because of this.					
16. Decisions are hard for me to make.					
17. I feel I need more rest and sleep.					
18. Family members think I should do more.					
19. I feel I need more privacy.					
20. I'm unable to get out to do what I need to.					
21. I'm embarrassed by my relative's behavior.					
22. I get easily upset with my relative.					
23. I feel I need more help.					
24. I feel I'm getting isolated.					
25. I'm afraid of what the future will be.					

Staff Stress Measure

This form is designed for use in nursing homes and day programs that care for Alzheimer's patients. For persons in supervisory and staff development positions, it can be useful in developing training programs and in working individually with employees. Direct care staff have the most contact with the Alzheimer's patient; therefore, they need a better understanding of the illness, how to deal with the behavior, and how to cope with this behavior emotionally. They need skills and sensitivity.

These staff in an open and supportive learning environment can be open and honest about their frustration and fears. They can also be receptive to suggestions when they begin to understand that the behavior of brain-impaired individuals can be more predictable and manageable.

STAFF STRESS MEASURE
DEMENTIA CARE

All statements below reflect feelings and beliefs that apply to work with residents who have Alzheimer's disease or a similar degenerative dementia. For each statement check how often you are affected in such a way.

	Rarely	Sometimes	Frequently	Nearly Always
1. Their forgetfulness really gets on my nerves.				
2. I believe these residents should do more for themselves.				
3. I'm afraid these residents will get violent and hurt someone.				
4. I get tired of repeating things to them so much.				
5. Their families just don't appreciate what we do for these people.				
6. Their babbling and rambling speech gets on my nerves.				
7. It's very hard for me to communicate with these people.				
8. I get mad when they deny problems and blame others for things.				
9. I really get tired working with these residents.				
10. It's hard to accept what is happening to these residents.				
11. I get frustrated and angry working with these people.				
12. I think more medication would make it easier to help them.				
13. I have trouble talking to their families.				
14. I take my work with them home with me.				
15. I feel these residents should appreciate our help more.				
16. It worries me these people will wander off.				
17. I feel it takes too long to do things for them.				
18. It bothers me how helpless these residents become.				
19. I believe we should have more training to work with them.				
20. It's difficult to explain their behavior to other residents or families.				

SERVICE/RESOURCE WORKSHEET

Name of agency: _____

Type of service/resource needed: _____

_____

What the service/resource will accomplish: _____

_____

Agency/individual providing service—contact person: _____

_____

Eligibility requirements (income, age, geographic): _____

_____

Fees/cost of service: _____

Projected cost of service over time: _____

Sliding scale for fee structure: _____

_____

Insurance coverage—how much, how long: _____

In-home and/or office services: _____

Benefit of service to family: _____

Other services provided by this agency: _____

_____

Providers recommended by professionals and/or friends: _____

_____

SERVICE/RESOURCE WORKSHEET
Example

Name of agency: *Home Health Care*

Type of service/resource needed: *Supervision of Alzheimer's patient in the home and assistance with basic personal care (bathing)*

What the service/resource will accomplish: *give caregiver time to get away, and do necessary errands, visit, shop*

Agency/individual providing service—contact person: *Home Health Care: Jodie Smith*

Eligibility requirements (income, age, geographic): *none for this type of service*

Fees/cost of service: *$5.00 an hour for 10 hours*

Projected cost of service over time: *about $200.00 a month times 12 months*

Sliding scale for fee structure: *none—different hourly rates for total monthly hours*

Insurance coverage—how much, how long: *none, unless nursing care needed*

In-home and/or office services: *All services provided in the home*

Benefit of service to family: *gives caregiver a break, time to do other things*

Other services provided by this agency: *Agency also has medical equipment, nursing services; occupational, physical, and speech therapists*

Providers recommended by professionals and/or friends: *This agency and Home Help Health Care (which is $8.00 an hour regardless)*

APPENDIX B
SELF-HELP GROUPS

A network of self-support groups exists through the Alzheimer's Disease and Related Disorders Association (ADRDA). Groups that have just become affiliated may not be listed here. There are also local support groups in some areas that are not affiliated with ADRDA. These groups may be helpful to the caregiver. To find out about a support group in your area, contact the Area Agency on Aging or the Information and Referral Program. ADRDA will have information about affiliated groups.

National Office—Alzheimer's Disease and Related Disorder Association, 70 East Lake Street, Suite 600, Chicago, IL 60601, 312-853-3060

Colorado

ADRDA-Denver, Rose Medical Center, 4567 East 9th Avenue, Denver, CO 80220, Janice DeTemple, 303-393-7675

District of Columbia

ADRDA-Metro Washington, 819 Aster Boulevard, Rockville, MD 20850, Helen Chambers, 301-424-9420

Florida

ADRDA-Greater Daytona Beach, 1282 Mayflower Drive, Daytona Beach, FL 32019, Mrs. Thomas K. Warke, 904-767-3757

ADRDA-Fort Myers (Lee County), Lee Mental Health Center, Inc., 2789 Ortiz Avenue, SE, P.O. Box 06137, Ft. Myers, FL 33906, Susan Workman or Suzanne Christ, 813-334-3537

ADRDA-Greater Jacksonville, 848 Glynlea Road, Jacksonville, FL 32216, Catherine Lester, 904-724-1447

ADRDA-Broward County (Florida), 9301 Sunrise Lake Boulevard, #109, Sunrise Lake, FL 33322, Eshter Rothchild, 305-741-3984

ADRDA-Manatee-Sarasota Counties, 6303 Sun Eagle Lane, Bradenton, FL 33507, Eva Davis, 813-755-4331; 585 Yawl Lane, Longboat Key, FL 33507, Bernice Braznell, 813-383-7870

Georgia

ADRDA-Atlanta, Wesley Woods Campus, 1817 Clifton Road, NE, Atlanta, GA 30029, Carolyn French, 404-633-8759; 4764 La Vista Road, Tucker, GA 30084, Martha Sanders, 404-491-8969

Hawaii

ADRDA-Honolulu Chapter, Inc., Ward Warehouse, Building D, Upper Level, 1050 Ala Moana Boulevard, Honolulu, HI 96816, Helen Mac-Bride, 808-521-3771

Illinois

ADRDA-Chicago, Eths, Room S-217, 1600 Dodge Street, Evanston, IL 60204, Carol Kallish, 312-864-0045

Indiana

ADRDA-St. Joseph County (South Bend, Indiana), 2113 Beverly Place, South Bend, IN 46616, Sadie Mager, 219-233-4444

Iowa

ADRDA-Des Moines, Iowa Methodist Medical Center, 1200 Pleasant Street, Des Moines, IA 50308, Linda Simonton, M.S.W., 515-283- 6431

Kansas

ADRDA-Greater Kansas City Area, 10108 West 96 Street, #B, Overland Park, KS 66212, Evelyn Sidner, 913-492-5228

Kentucky

ADRDA-Louisville, 6607 Watch Hill Road, Louisville, KY 40228, Ed Schmidt, 502-239-9329

Maryland

ADRDA-Baltimore, P.O. Box 9751, Baltimore, MD 21204, Glenn Kirkland, 301-792-7800, ext. 7224

Massachusetts

ADRDA-Massachusetts, Boston University School of Medicine, 80 East Concord Street, Boston, MA 02118, F. Marrott Sinex, Ph.D., 617-247-5941

Michigan

ADRDA-Greater Ann Arbor, 1225 Astor Drive, #222, Ann Arbor, MI 48104, Alma L. Ford, 313-662-6638

ADRDA-Detroit, 725 S. Adams, Suite L-6, Birmingham, MI 48011, Nancy Lombardo or Sarah Glover, 313-540-2373 or 313-332-4110

ADRDA-Flint & Genessee County, 514 East Main Street, Flushing, MI 48433, John Tomaszweksi, 313-659-4435

ADRDA-Grand Rapids Area (Serving West Michigan), P.O. Box 1646, Grand Rapids, MI 49505, General Information 616-245-5735; Elly Lenihan, 616-456-5664; Michael L. Hale, 616-243-0231

ADRDA-Mid-Michigan, 9470 Rosebush Road, Mt. Pleasant, MI 48858, Mary Spierling, 517-465-6602

Minnesota

ADRDA-Association for Alzheimer's and Related Diseases, 2501 West 84 Street, Bloomington, MN 55431, Audrey Lindahl, 612-888-7653

Missouri

ADRDA-St. Louis, Washington University, School of Medicine, P.O. Box 8111, 660 S. Euclid Avenue, St. Louis, MO 63310, Warren Danziger, Ph.D., 314-454-2384

Nebraska

ADRDA-Lincoln, 4600 Valley Road, Lincoln, NE 68510, Marilyn Baalhorn, 402-489-6513

ADRDA-Omaha, P.O. Box 14933, Omaha, NE 68124, Cheryl McKay, 402- 334-0506; Ralph Peppard, 402-399-9069

Nevada

ADRDA-Las Vegas, Charleston Convalescent Center, 2035 Charleston Boulevard, Las Vegas, NV 89102, Janna Benkelman, 702-386-7980

New Mexico

ADRDA-Albuquerque, 1027 Pampas Drive, SE, Albuquerque, NM 87108, Nance Dancy, 505-299-8223; Marian Knapp, 505-266-6621

New York

ADRDA-Capital District (Albany), 87 Brookline Avenue, Albany, NY 12203, Barbara Vickers, 518-438-4929

ADRDA-Alzheimer's Disease Society, 32 West Broadway, New York, NY 10004, Lonnie E. Wollin, Esq., Mailing Address: 1435 Tenth Street, Ft. Lee, NJ 07024, 212-736-3670 or 201-224-0388

ADRDA-Manhattan, 125 West 76th Street, New York, NY 10023 ADRDA-Nassau and Suffolk Counties, 579 Monroe Street, Cedarhurst, NY 11516, Ellen Tolle, 516-569-2310

ADRDA-Rochester, 24 Harvard Street, Rochester, NY 14607, Jim Reveley, 716-473-1634(H) or 716-442-3820

ADRDA-Westchester, 785 Mamaroneck, White Plains, NY 10605, Renee Pollack or Marilyn Herman, 914-428-1919

ADRDA-Western New York (located in the Buffalo area), Dent Neurological Institute, Millard Fillmore Hospital, 3 Gate Circle, Buffalo, NY 14209, Barbara Galus, 716-873-2988

North Carolina

ADRDA-Duke Family Support Network, Room 153, Civitan Building, Duke University Medical Center, Durham, NC 27710, Lisa Gwyther, 919-684-2328

Ohio

ADRDA-Athens, 37 Pleasant View Drive, Athens, OH 45701, Dr. Anne Samaan, 614-592-2013(H) or 614-592-1913(W)

ADRDA-Canton, 1509 Howenstine Drive, SE, East Sparta, OH 44626, Lynn Wasnak, 216-484-5878

ADRDA-Cincinnati, 8995 Tripoli Drive, Cincinnati, OH 45239, Elizabeth Bolles, 513-729-3271

ADRDA-Cleveland, 1801 Chestnut Hills Drive, Cleveland, OH 44106, Carolyn Lookabill, 216-721-8457

ADRDA-Alzheimer's Disease Association, Martin Janis Senior Center, 600 East 11 Avenue, Columbus, OH 43211, Dr. Gerland Robinson, 614-299-2327

ADRDA-Dayton Area, 157 Shenandoah Trail, West Carrollton, OH 45449, Doris Palm, 513-435-0151

ADRDA-Youngstown, 344 S. Broad Street, Canfield, OH 44406, Diana Williams, 216-533-7234

Oklahoma

ADRDA-Oklahoma City Area Chapter, 1613 Andover Ct., Oklahoma City, OK 73120, Jerry Robinson, 405-843-4680

Oregon

ADRDA-Columbia-Williamette (located in the Portland area), Neurological Sciences Center, Good Samaritan Hospital, 1015 NW 22 Avenue, Portland, OR 97210, Sharon Moody, 503-232-0306

Pennsylvania

ADRDA-Cobs, 1201 Arrott Building, 401 Wood Street, Pittsburgh, PA 15222, Martha Fenchak Bell, 412-355-5248 or 412-469-1567

ADRDA-Greater Philadelphia, 821 Clifford Avenue, Ardmore, PA 19003, Peggy Morscheck, 215-649-3198; George Bates, 215-485-4528, or 2424 Easton, #D3, Willow Grove, PA 19090, Ed Mello, 215-441-4614

Rhode Island

ADRDA-Providence, Gerontology Center, Rhode Island College, 600 Mt. Pleasant Avenue, Providence, RI 02908, Sylvia Zaki, 401-456- 8276

Tennessee

ADRDA-Memphis, 4060 Southlawn Avenue, Memphis, TN 38111, Dot King, 901-744-1165

Texas

ADRDA-Amarillo, Route 6, Box 760, Amarillo, TX 79106, Becky McGee, 806-381-1010

ADRDA-Dallas, 11216 Dumbarton, Dallas, TX 75228, Jo Ann Ray, 214-270-9604(H) or 214-948-7973(W)

ADRDA-El Paso, 6545 Fiesta Drive, El Paso, TX 79912, Grace Braly, 915-581-4926

ADRDA-Tarrant County (Forth Worth), 2925 Conejos Drive, Fort Worth, TX 76116, Bill Walters, 817-244-1085

ADRDA-Houston, 8101 Amelia, #304C, Houston, TX 77055, Lois Mullen, 713-465-9505(H) or 713-869-5546(W)

Utah

ADRDA-Greater Ogden, 232 Polk Avenue, Ogden, UT 84404, Pat Sackett, 801-392-5588

Virginia

ADRDA-Hampton Roads, Comprehensive Mental Health Service, Pembroke Three, Suite 109, Virginia Beach, VA 23462, Terry Jenkins, 804-490-0583

ADRDA-Northern Virginia, P.O. Box 2715, Springfield, VA 22152, John Dingle, 703-273-5453

ADRDA-Richmond, Counseling & Psychological Services, P.O. Box 3185, Richmond, VA 23235, Nan Wentzel, 804-794-9723, or 1163 Southam Drive, Richmond, VA 23235, Paul Gerhardt, 804-320-3365

ADRDA-Roanoke/Salem, VA Medical Center, Salem, VA 24153, Jean Taylor, 703-982-2463, ext. 2477

Wisconsin
ADRDA-Greater Milwaukee, Wisconsin Regional Geriatric Center, Family Hospital, 2711 West Wells Street, Milwaukee, WI 53208, Barbara Keyes, 414-933-6769; Dorothy Heydinger, 414-547-6406

AREA AGENCIES ON AGING

Area Agencies on Aging carry out implementation of programs for older persons that are indicated by the Older American's Act. The Administration on Aging has this responsibility at the federal level. Area Agencies on Aging are a local extension of the federal agency. Usually there is a state Department on Aging that governs Area Agencies on Aging for each state. The reader may call the State Department on Aging to determine what Area Agency on Aging covers his particular location.

Administration on Aging
330 Independence Avenue
Washington, DC 20201
General Information: 202-472-7257

Alabama
Commission on Aging, 502 Washington Avenue, Montgomery, AL 36130; 205-261-5743

Alaska
Older Alaskans Commission, Department of Administration, Pouch C-MS-0209, Juneau, AK 99811; 907-465-3250

Arizona
Office on Aging and Adult Administration, P.O. Box 6123, 1400 West Washington Street, Phoenix, AZ 85007; 602-255-3596

Arkansas
Division of Aging and Adult Services, Donaghey Building, Suite 1428, 7th and Main Street, Little Rock, AR 72201; 501-371-2441

California
Department of Aging, 1600 K Street, Sacramento, CA 95814; 916-322-5290

Colorado

Aging and Adult Services Division, Department of Social Services, 717 17th Street, P.O. Box 181000, Denver, CO 80218-0899; 303-294-5913

Connecticut

Department on Aging, 175 Main Street, Hartford, CT 06106; 203-566-3238

Delaware

Department of Health and Social Services, Division of Aging, 1901 North Dupont Highway, New Castle, DE 19720; 302-421-6791

District of Columbia

Office of Aging, 1424 K Street, N.W., Washington, DC 20011; 202-724-5626

Florida

Aging and Adult Services, Department of Health and Rehabilitative Services, 1317 Winewood Boulevard, Tallahassee, FL 32301; 904-488-8922

Georgia

Office of Aging, 878 Peachtree Street, N.E., Room 632, Atlanta, GA 30309; 404-894-5333

Hawaii

Executive Office on Aging, Office of the Governor, State of Hawaii, Room 241, 335 Merchant Street, Honolulu, HI 96813, 808-548-2593

Idaho

Idaho Office on Aging, Statehouse Room 114, Boise, ID 83720; 208-334-3833

Illinois

Illinois Department on Aging, 421 East Capitol Avenue, Springfield, IL 62701; 217-785-2870

Indiana

Indiana Department on Aging and Community Services, 251 North Illinois Street, P.O. Box 7083, Indianapolis, IN 46207-7083; 317-232-7006

Iowa

Department of Elder Affairs, Suite 236, Jewett Building, 914 Grand Avenue, Des Moines, IA 50319; 515-281-5187

Kansas

Kansas Department of Aging, 610 West 10th Street, Topeka, KS 66612; 913-296-4986

Kentucky
Kentucky Division for Aging Services, Department of Human Resources, DHR Building-6th Floor, 275 East Main Street, Frankfort, KY 40601; 502-564-6930

Louisiana
Louisiana Office of Elderly Affairs, P.O. Box 80374, Capital Station, Baton Rouge, LA 70898; 504-925-1700

Maine
Bureau of Maine's Elderly, Department of Human Services, State House Station 11, Augusta, ME 04333; 207-289-2561

Maryland
Maryland Office on Aging, State Office Building, 301 West Preston Street, Baltimore, MD 21201; 301-225-1100

Massachusetts
Executive Office of Elder Affairs, 38 Chauncey Street, Boston, MA 02111; 617-727-7750

Michigan
Michigan Office of Services to the Aging, 300 East Michigan, P.O. Box 30026, Lansing, MI 48909; 517-373-8230

Minnesota
Minnesota Board on Aging, 204 Metro Square Building, Seventh and Robert Street, St. Paul, MN 55101; 612-296-2544

Mississippi
Mississippi Council on Aging, 301 West Pearl Street, Jackson, MS 39203-3092; 601-949-2070

Missouri
Missouri Office of Aging, Department of Social Services, 2701 West Main Street, Jefferson City, MO 65102; 314-751-3082

Montana
Community Services Division, Department of Social and Rehabilitation Services, P.O. Box 4210, Helena, MT 59604; 406-444-3865

Nebraska
Nebraska Department on Aging, P.O. Box 95044, 301 Centennial Mall South, Lincoln, NE 68509; 402-471-2306

Nevada
Division of Aging Services, Department of Human Resources, 505 East King Street, Room 101, Kinkead Building, Carson City, NV 89710; 702-885-4210

New Hampshire

New Hampshire Council on the Aging, 105 Loudon Road-Bldg. #3, Concord, NH 03301; 603-271-2751

New Jersey

Division on Aging, Department of Community Affairs, P.O. Box 2768, 363 West State Street, Trenton, NJ 08625; 609-292-4833

New Mexico

New Mexico State Agency on Aging, La Villa Rivera Building, 224 East Palace Avenue, Santa Fe, NM 87501; 505-827-7640

New York

Office for the Aging, New York State Executive Department, Agency Building 2, Empire State Plaza, Albany, NY 12223; 518-474-5731

North Carolina

Division on Aging, Department of Human Resources, 1985 Umpstead Dr.-Kirby Bldg., Raleigh, NC 27603; 919-733-3983

North Dakota

Aging Services, Department of Human Services, State Capital Building, Bismark, ND 58505; 701-224-2577

Ohio

Ohio Department on Aging, Ninth Floor, 50 West Broad Street, Columbus, OH 43215; 614-466-5500

Oklahoma

Special Unit on Aging, Department of Human Services, P.O. Box 25352, Oklahoma City, OK 73125; 405-521-2281

Oregon

Senior Services Division, Human Resources Department, Room 313, Public Services Building, Salem, OR 97301; 503-378-4728

Pennsylvania

Pennsylvania Department of Aging, 231 State Street, Harrisburg, PA 17101; 717-783-1550

Rhode Island

Department of Elderly Affairs, 79 Washington Street, Providence, RI 02903; 401-277-2858

South Carolina

South Carolina Commission of Aging, 915 Main Street, Columbia, SC 29201; 803-783-3203

South Dakota
Office of Adult Services and Aging, Division of Human Development, Department of Social Services, Richard F. Kneip Building, 700 North Illinois Street, Pierre, SD 57501; 605-773-3656

Tennessee
Tennessee Commission on Aging, Suite 201, 706 Church Street, Nashville, TN 37219-5573; 615-741-2056

Texas
Texas Department of Aging, P.O. Box 12786, Capital Station, 1949 IH 35 South, Austin, TX 78711; 512-444-2727

Utah
Division of Aging and Adult Services, Department of Social Services, 150 West North Temple, Salt Lake City, UT 84145-0500; 801-533-6422

Vermont
Vermont Office on the Aging, 103 South Main Street, Waterbury, VT 05676; 803-241-2400

Virginia
Virginia Department on Aging, 101 North 14th Street-18th Floor, James Monroe Bldg., Richmond, VA 23219; 804-225-2271

Washington
Aging and Adult Services Administration, Department of Social and Health Services, OB-44B, Olympia, WA 98504; 206-586-3768

West Virginia
Commission on Aging, Holly Grove-State Capitol, Charleston, WV 25305; 304-348-3317

Wisconsin
Bureau of Aging, Division of Community Services, Room 480, 1 West Wilson Street, Madison, WI 53702; 608-266-2536

Wyoming
Commission on Aging, Room 139, Hathaway Building, Cheyenne, WY 82002; 307-777-7986

AN AFTERWORD

When I was about 17, I found an old German drinking mug hidden among the rubble heaped along a creek near my grandparents' home in an isolated rural area near Waco, Texas. The creek, one of my favorite places, was exciting to explore, partly because I could hide in the sea cane and splash through the water, but also because I always hoped I would find something ancient and valuable there. My eyes alert for old coins and arrowheads, I would find instead rusty cans and buckles from old mule harnesses—until the day I spotted the old mug. The handle was broken, but as with many decorative mugs of its type, there were inscriptions on it in old German. Surely, I thought, there was some great truth revealed there, if only I could find someone to translate it.

My family had long since stopped speaking German and had largely forgotten the language, but I searched for someone to help me understand what the words meant. Finally, a high school German teacher found someone to translate the ancient German saying:

> God protect you.
> Things have happened
> Differently than I imagined

> and

> God protect you.
> It would have been nice.

In my adolescent frame of mind, I thought at the time the inscription must have related to a long-ago youth who had lost his first love. Later when I began working with the elderly and their families, how-ever, that saying deepened in meaning with an application to losses of a very different nature. It is hard to accept lost dreams, unfulfilled at the end of a brief romance. It is quite another thing to see plans and dreams made over decades slowly but unrelentingly ripped apart by an illness that seems to go on forever before it ends.

The ancient saying takes on new meaning when I look at it today, applying those words to the people I work with daily—victims of Alzheimer's and their families, engaged in a long good-bye filled with the acceptance of something that is not over, at least not yet.

I remember how the mug had been chipped in a number of places, the porcelain finish cracked from the ravages of time and weather. As a teenager, I imagined how beautiful the mug must have been long ago. I thought of all the history it could have shared with me if it could have talked. Many times, I tried to find ways to restore the mug to its original condition. The chips were filled in, but that did not help much. It was still chipped and could not be restored.

Finally, I accepted the mug for what it was. It was still special, and the message it carried became more meaningful as time passed. I could not put the mug back into its original shape. Its personal value to me cannot be fully appreciated by others. Its original function and purpose has been lost, but it still occupies an honorable place on a bookshelf in my home, and its message serves to remind me that life is full of losses and disappointments, but it is also full of hopes.

It is common to look back on what has happened, the good and the bad, when we have lost someone. In the case of Alzheimer's, your caregiving made a difference to the one you loved. You need to hear that now, to accept it, and to let it make a difference to you.

Any one of us could say that things have worked out differently than we imagined. If we are thinking of only what could have been, we are probably pondering how nice it could have been. We might ponder instead what was and still is—the experiences, the memories, and the accomplishments of one's whole life. And they are nice, too, aren't they?

Behut dich Gott,
(God Protect You)

Howard Gruetzner
Waco, Texas

BIBLIOGRAPHY

Agbayewa, O.M. "Earlier Psychiatric Morbidity in Patients with Alzheimer's Disease." *JAGS*, *34* (1986):561–564.

Appel, S.H., and McManaman, L. "Is a Breakdown of the Blood-Brain Barrier Cause or Effect?" *Neurobiology of Aging*, *7* (1986):512–574.

Bajada. "A Trial of Choline Chloride and Physostigmine in Alzheimer's Dementia." *Alzheimer's Disease: A Report of Progress in Research (Aging*, Vol. 19), edited by Corkin, S. et al., 427–432. New York: Raven Press, 1982.

Ball, M.J. "Granulovacuolar Degeneration." In *Alzheimer's Disease: The Standard Reference*, edited by Reisberg, B., 62–68. New York: The Free Press, 1983.

Ball, M.J. et al. "A New Definition of Alzheimer's Disease: A Hippocampal Dementia." *The Lancet* (January 5, 1985):14–16.

Barnes, D.M. "Defect in Alzheimer's Is on Chromosome 21." *Science, 235* (1987):846–847.

Bartus, R.T. "Effects of Cholinergic Agents on Learning and Memory in Animal Models of Aging." *Alzheimer's Disease: A Report of Progress in Research (Aging*, Vol. 19), edited by Corkin, S. et al., 271–280. New York: Raven Press, 1982.

Bartus, R.T. et al. "The Cholinergic Hypothesis of Geriatric Memory Dysfunction." *Science, 217* (1982):408–417.

Beal, M.F. et al. "Reduced Numbers of Somatostatin Receptors in the Cerebral Cortex in Alzheimer's Disease." *Science, 229* (1985):289–291.

Beaumont, J.G. *Introduction to Neuropsychology*. New York: The Gullford Press, 1983.

Behan, P.O., and Behan, Wm. H. "Possible Immunological Factors in Alzheimer's Disease." In *Alzheimer's Disease: Early Recognition of Potentially Reversible Deficits*, edited by Glen A.I.M., and Whalley, L.J., 33–35. Edinburgh, London, and New York: Churchill Livingstone, 1979.

Belza, M.G., and Urich, H. "Cerebral Amyloid Angiopathy in Down's Syndrome." *Clinical Neuropathology, 5*, no. 6 (1986):257–260.

Berg, L. "Aging and Dementia." In *Neurological Pathophysiology*, edited by Pearlman, A.L., and Collins, R.C., 250–273. New York: Oxford University Press, 1984.

Bjorklund, A. et al. "Intracerebral Neural Grafting in Animal Models of Aging Brain: Strategies, Rationale, and Preliminary Results." *DMB, Gerontology, 1* (1985):35–39.

231

Blackwood, O.H.R., and Christie, J.E. "The Effects of Physostigmine on Memory and Auditory p 300 in Alzheimer-Type Dementia." *Biol. Psychiatry, 21* (1986):557–560.

Blass, J.P. et al. "To the Editor." *New England Journal of Medicine* (1983):309.

Bloom, T.E. et al. *Brain, Mind, and Behavior.* New York: W.H. Freeman and Company, 1985.

Bondareff, W. "Age and Alzheimer's Disease." *The Lancet* (June 25, 1983):1447.

Bondareff, W. "Biomedical Perspective of Alzheimer's Disease and Dementia in the Elderly." In *The Dementias: Policy and Management,* edited by Gilhooly M.L.M. et al., 13–37. New Jersey: Prentice-Hall, 1986.

Bondareff, W. et al. "Quantitative Computed Tomography in Senile Dementia." *Arch. Gen. Psychiatry, 38* (1981):1365–1368.

Bondareff, W. et al. "Loss of Neurons of Origin of the Adrenergic Projection to Cerebral Cortex (nucleus locus coeruleus) in Senile Dementia." *Neurology, 32* (1982):164–168.

Bowen, D.M. "Neurochemical Findings in Alzheimer's Disease." In *Alzheimer's Disease Early Recognition of Potentially Reversible Deficits,* edited by Glen, A.I.M., and Whalley, L.J., 17–26. London and New York: Churchill Livingstone, 1979.

Breitner, J.C.S., and Folstein, M.F. "Familial Alzheimer Dementia: A Prevalent Disorder with Specific Clinical Features." *Psychiatric Medicine, 14* (1984):63–80.

Brinkman, S.D., and Largen, J.W., Jr. "Strategies for the Pharmacological Treatment of Alzheimer's Disease." *Texas Medicine, 83* (1987):26–30.

Brun, A. "An Overview of Light and Electron Microscopic Changes." In *Alzheimer's Disease: The Standard Reference,* edited by Reisberg, B., 37–48. New York: The Free Press, 1983.

Brun, A. "The Structural Development of Alzheimer's Disease." *DMB, Gerontology, 1* (1985):25–27.

Bruno, G. et al. "Muscarinic Agonist Therapy of Alzheimer's Disease." *Arch. Neurol., 43* (1986):459–661.

Cardelli, M.B. et al. "Chelation Therapy. Unproved Modality in the Treatment of Alzheimer-Type Dementia." *J. Am. Geriatr. Soc., 33* (1985):548–551.

Carlsson, A. "Changes in Neurotransmitter Systems in the Aging Brain and in Alzheimer's Disease." In *Alzheimer's Disease: The Standard Reference,* edited by Reisberg, B., 100–106. New York: The Free Press, 1983.

Carlsson, A. "Neurotransmitter Changes in the Aging Brain." *DMB, Gerontology, 1* (1985):40–43.

Carter, C.J. "Selective Loss of Neurons of Origin of Adrenergic Projection to Cerebral Cortex (Nucleus Locus Coeruleus) in Senile Dementia." *The Lancet* (April 4, 1982):783–784.

Chase. T.N. et al. "Vasopressin Treatment of Cognitive Deficits in Alzheimer's Disease." *Alzheimer's Disease: A Report of Progress in Research (Aging,* Vol. 19), edited by Corkin, S. et al., 457–462. New York: Raven Press, 1982.

Check, W. "Forebrain Yields Clues to Alzheimer's Disease." *JAMA, 249,* no. 15 (1983):1975–1979.

Christie, J.E. "Neurophysiology of Dementia." In *Alzheimer's Disease: Early Recognition of Potentially Reversible Deficits*, edited by Glen, A.I.M., and Whalley, L.J., 163-168. London and New York: Churchill Livingstone, 1979.

Christie, J.E. "Physostigmine and Arecoline Infusions in Alzheimer's Disease." In *Alzheimer's Disease: A Report of Progress in Research (Aging*, Vol. 19), edited by Corkin, S. et al., 413-420. New York: Raven Press, 1982.

Chui, H.C. et al. "Clinical Subtypes of Dementia of the Alzheimer's type." *Neurology, 35* (1985):1544-1550.

Cohen, D., and Eisdorfer, C. *The Loss of Self: A Family Resource for the Care of Alzheimer's Disease and Related Disorders.* New York: W.W. Norton and Company, 1986.

Conley, Charles, M.D. Personal communication with author, July, 1987.

Constantinidis, J. "Is Alzheimer's Disease a Major Form of Senile Dementia? Clinical Anatomical and Genetic Data." In *Alzheimer's Disease: Senile Dementia and Related Disorders (Aging*, Vol. 7), edited by Katzman, R. et al., 15-26. New York: Raven Press, 1978.

Constantinidis, J. "Zinc Metabolism in presenile dementias." In *Alzheimer's Disease: Early Recognition of Potentially Reversible Deficits*, edited by Glen A.I.M., and Whalley, L.J., 48-50. London and New York: Churchill Livingstone, 1979.

Cooper, S.J. "Drug Treatments, Neurochemical Change and Human Memory Impairment." In *Clinical Management of Memory Problems*, edited by Wilson, Barbara, and Moffat, Nick, 132-147. London: Aspen Publication, 1984.

Corsellis, J.A.N. "Post-traumatic Dementia." In *Alzheimer's Disease: Senile Dementia and Related Disorders (Aging*, Vol. 7), edited by Katzman, R. et al., 125-135. New York: Raven Press, 1978.

Corser, C.M. et al. "Effect of Lecithin in Senile Dementia: A report of four cases." In *Alzheimer's Disease: Early Recognition of Potentially Reversible Deficits*, edited by Glen A.I.M., and Whalley, L.J., 169-172. London and New York: Churchill Livingstone, 1979.

Coyle, J.T. et al. "Alzheimer's Disease: A Disorder of Cortical Cholinergic Innervation." *Science, 219* (1983):1184-1189.

Crapper, D.R. et al. "Aluminum and Other Metals in Senile (Alzheimer) Dementia." In *Alzheimer's Disease: Senile Dementia and Related Disorders (Aging*, Vol. 7), edited by Katzman, R. et al., 471-486. New York: Raven Press, 1978.

Cummings, J.L. "Organic Delusions: Phenomenology, Anatomical Correlations, and Review." *Brit. J. Psychia., 146* (1985):184-197.

Cummings, J.L. "Subcortical Dementia: Neuropsychology, Neuropsychiatry, and Pathophysiology." *Brit. J. Psychia., 149* (1986):682-697.

Cummings, J.L. "Dementia Syndromes: Neurobehavioral and Neuropsychiatric Features." *J. Clin. Psychiatry, 48* (1987):3-8.

Cummings, J.L., and Benson, D.F. *Dementia: A Clinical Approach.* Boston: Butterworths, 1983, 35-167.

Cummings, J.L., and Benson, D.F. "Subcortical Dementia." *Arch. Neurol., 41* (1984):874-879.

Cummings, J.L. et al. "Aphasia in Dementia of the Alzheimer's Type." *Neurology, 35* (1985):394–397.

Cummings, J.L., and Benson, D.F. "Dementia of the Alzheimer Type, An inventory of Diagnostic Clinical Features." *JAGS, 34* (1986):12–19.

Cutler, R.W.P. "Degenerative and Hereditary Diseases." *Scientific Amer., 11* (1984):1–13.

Davamand, D.P., and Nelson, J.C. "Concurrent Depression and Dementia: Implications for Diagnosis and Treatment." *J. Clin. Psychiatry, 46* (1985):389–392.

Davies, B.M. et al. "Clinical Studies of the Cholinergic Deficit in Alzheimer's Disease." *JAGS, 33,* no. 11 (1985):741–747.

Davies, P. "Studies on the Neurochemistry of Central Cholinergic Systems in Alzheimer's Disease." In *Alzheimer's Disease: Senile Dementia and Related Disorders (Aging,* Vol. 7), edited by Katzman, R. et al., 453–460. New York: Raven Press, 1978.

Davies, P. "The Genetics of Alzheimer's Disease: A Review and a Discussion of the Implications." *Neuro. Aging, 7* (1986):459–466.

Davies, P., Katz, D.A., and Crystal, H.A. "Choline Acetyltransferase, Somatostatin, and Substance P in Selected Cases of Alzheimer's Disease." In *Alzheimer's Disease: A Report of Progress in Research (Aging,* Vol. 19), edited by Corkin, S. et al., 9–14. New York: Raven Press, 1982.

Davies, P., and Wolozin, B.L. "Recent Advances in the Neurochemistry of Alzheimer's Disease." *J. Clin. Psychiatry, 48* (1987):23–30.

Davis, K.L. et al. "Cholinergic Treatment in Alzheimer's Disease: Implications for Future Research." In *Alzheimer's Disease: A Report of Progress in Research (Aging,* Vol. 19), edited by Corkin, S. et al., 483–494. New York: Raven Press, 1982.

Delabar, J.M. et al."B Amyloid Gene Duplication in Alzheimer's Disease and Karyotypically Normal Down Syndrom." *Science, 235* (1987):1390–1392.

Diagnostic and Statistical Manual of Mental Disorders, Third Edition. 1980. Washington, D.C.: American Psychiatric Association, 101–128.

Domino, E.F. et al. "Effects of Oral Lecithin on Both Blood Choline Levels and Memory Tests in Geriatric Volunteers." In *Alzheimer's Disease: A Report of Progress in Research (Aging,* Vol. 19), edited by Corkin, S. et al., 393–398. New York: Raven Press, 1982.

Drachman, D.A. "Memory, Dementia, and the Cholinergic System." In *Alzheimer's Disease: Senile Dementia and Related Disorders (Aging,* Vol. 7), edited by Katzman, R. et al., 143–150. New York: Raven Press, 1978.

Drachman, D.A. "The Pharmacologic Basis for Cholinergic Investigations of Alzheimer's Disease: Evidence and Implications." In *Alzheimer's Disease: A Standard Reference,* edited by Reisberg, B., 340–345. New York: The Free Press, 1983.

Dunn, A., and Brody, S. *Functional Chemistry of the Brain.* New York: Spectrum Publications, 1974.

Dysken, M.W. "A Review of Recent Clinical Trials in the Treatment of Alzheimer's Dementia." *Psychiatric Annals, 17* (1987): 178–191.

Dysken, M.W. et al. "Lecithin Administration in Alzheimer Dementia." *Neuro., 32* (1982):1203–1204.

Dysken, M.W., Tovall, P. et al. "Lecithin Administration in Patients with Primary Degenerative Dementia and in Normal volunteers." In *Alzheimer's Disease: A Report of Progress in Research (Aging,* Vol. 19), edited by Corkin, S. et al., 385–392. New York: Raven Press, 1982.

Eastham, J. et al. "Caregivers for Dementia Patients: A Comparison of Husbands and wives." *The Gerontologist, 26* (1986).

Editorial. "Cholinergic Treatment in Alzheimer's Disease: Encouraging Results." *The Lancet* (Jan. 17, 1987):139–141.

Edmond, E. "Conventional viruses in slow infection of the central nervous system." In *Alzheimer's Disease: Early Recognition of Potentially Reversible Deficits,* edited by Glen A.I.M., and Whalley, L.J., 46–48. London and New York: Churchill Livingstone, 1979.

Edye, D., and Rich, J. *Psychological Distress in Aging: A Family Management Model.* Rockville, Maryland: Aspen Publication, 1986.

Etienne, P. "Treatment of Alzheimer's Disease with Lecithin." In *Alzheimer's Disease: The Standard Reference,* edited by Reisberg, B., 353–354. New York: The Free Press, 1983.

Etienne, P. et al. "Alzheimer's Disease: Clinical Effect of Lecithin Treatment." In *Alzheimer's Disease: Early Recognition of Potentially Reversible Deficits,* edited by Glen A.I.M., and Whalley, L.J., 173–178. London and New York: Churchill Livingstone, 1979.

Etienne, P. et al. "Lecithin in the Treatment of Alzheimer's Disease." In *Alzheimer's Disease: A Report of Progress in Research (Aging,* Vol. 19), edited by Corkin, S. et al., 369–372. New York: Raven Press, 1982.

Faden, A.I., and Townsend, J.J. "Myoclonus in Alzheimer's Disease." *Arch. Neurol., 33* (1976):278–280.

Fann, W.E., and Wheless, J.C. "Treatment and Amelioration of Psychopathologic Affective States in the Dementias of Late Life." In *Clinical Aspects of Alzheimer's Disease and Senile Dementia (Aging,* Vol. 15), edited by Miller, N.E., and Cohen, G.D., 161–186. New York: Raven Press, 1981.

Ferris, S.H. "Neuropeptides in the Treatment of Alzheimer's Disease. In *Alzheimer's Disease: The Standard Reference,* edited by Reisberg, B., 369–373. New York: The Free Press, 1983.

Ferris, S.H. et al. "Pharmacologic Treatment of Senile Dementia: Choline, L-Dopa, Piracetam, and Choline Plus Piracetam." In *Alzheimer's Disease: A Report of Progress in Research (Aging,* Vol. 19), edited by Corkin, S. et al., 475–482. New York: Raven Press, 1982.

Fillit, H.M. et al. "Antivascular Antibodies in the Sera of Patients with Senile Dementia of the Alzheimer's Type." *J. Gerontology, 42* (1987):180–184.

Fine, A. "Transplantation in the Central Nervous System." *Scien. Amer., 255* (1986): 52–59.

Fischman, H.K. "Chromosomal factors." In *Alzheimer's Disease: The Standard Reference,* edited by Reisberg, B., 161–165. New York: The Free Press, 1983.

Folstein, M.F., and Breitner, J.C.S. "Language Disorder Predicts Familial Alzheimer's Disease." In *Alzheimer's Disease: A Report of Progress in Research (Aging,* Vol. 19), edited by Corkin, S. et al., 197–200. New York: Raven Press, 1982.

Folstein, M.F., and McHugh, P.R. "Dementia Syndrome of Depression." In *Alzheimer's Disease: Senile Dementia and Related Disorders (Aging,* Vol. 7), edited by Katzman, R. et al., 87–93. New York: Raven Press, 1978.

Folstein, M.F. et al. "The Meaning of Cognitive Impairment in the Elderly." *JAGS, 33* (1985):228–235.

Fovall, P., Dysken, M.W., and Davis, J.M. "Treatment of Alzheimer's Disease with Choline Salts." In *Alzheimer's Disease: The Standard Reference,* edited by Reisberg, B., 346–353. New York: The Free Press, 1983.

Francis, P.T. et al. "Neurochemical Studies of Early-onset Alzheimer's Disease." *N. Engl. J. Med., 313* (1985):7–11.

Fry, P.S. *Depression, Stress and Adaptations in the Elderly: Psychological Assessment and Intervention.* Rockville, Maryland: Aspen Publications, 1986.

Funkenstein, H.H. et al. "Drug Treatment of Cognitive Impairment in Alzheimer's Disease and the Late Life Dementias." *Clinical Aspects of Alzheimer's Disease and Senile Dementia (Aging,* Vol. 15), edited by Miller, N.E., and Cohen, G.D., 139–160. New York: Raven Press, 1981.

Gage, F.H. et al. "Intrahippocampal Septal Grafts Ameliorate Learning Impairments in Aged Rats." *Science,* (1984):533–536.

Gambetti, P. et al. "Paired Helical Filaments: Do They Contain Neurofilament Epitopes?" *Neurobiology of Aging, 7* (1986):451–452.

Gash, D.M. et al. "Neuronal Transplantation: A Review of Recent Developments and Potential Applications to the Aged Brain." *Neurobiology of Aging, 6* (1985):131–150.

George, L.K., and Gwyther, L.P. "Caregiver Well-being: A Multidimensional Examination of Family Caregivers of Demented Adults." *The Gerontologist, 26* (1986):3.

Gillin, J.C. "Cholinergic Mechanisms in Human Memory." In *Alzheimer's Disease: Early Recognition of Potentially Reversible Deficits,* edited by Glen A.I.M., and Whalley, L.J., 159–162. London and New York: Churchill Livingstone, 1979.

Glen, A.I.M. "Choice of Therapeutic Agents in Alzheimer's Disease." In *Alzheimer's Disease: Early Recognition of Potentially Reversible Deficits,* edited by Glen A.I.M., and Whalley, L.J., 140–148. London and New York: Churchill Livingstone, 1979.

Glen, A.I.M., and Christie, J.E. "Early Recognition of Alzheimer's Disease: Working Definitions for Clinical and Laboratory Criteria." In *Alzheimer's Disease: Early Recognition of Potentially Reversible Deficits,* edited by Glen A.I.M., and Whalley, L.J., 122–128. London and New York: Churchill Livingstone, 1979.

Glenner, G.G. "Amyloid Deposits and Amyloidosis." *N. Engl. J. Med., 302* (1980):1283–1292.

Glenner, G.G. "Amyloid Deposits and Amyloidosis." *N. Engl. J. Med., 302* (1980):1333–1343.

Glenner, G.G. "Current Knowledge of Amyloid Deposits as Applied to Senile Plaques and Congophilic Angiopathy." In *Alzheimer's Disease: Senile Dementia and Related Disorders (Aging,* Vol. 7), edited by Katzman, R. et al., 493–501. New York: Raven Press, 1978.

Goldgaber, D. et al. "Characterization and Chromosomal Localization of a cDNA Encoding Brain Amyloid of Alzheimer's Disease." *Science, 235* (1987):877–880.

Goldman, L.S., and Luchins, J. "Depression in the Spouse of Demented Patients." *Am. J. Psychiatry, 144* (1984):1467–1468.

Goldsmith, M.F. "Attempts to Vanquish Alzheimer's Disease Intensify, Take New Paths." *JAMA, 251* (1984):1805–1807, 1811–1812.

Gottfries, C.G. "Neurotransmitters in the brains of patients with dementia disorders." *DMB, Gerontology, 1* (1985):44–47.

Gottfries, C.G. "Is Alzheimer's a Homogenous Disease, Are Plaques Critical and Does the Blood Brain Barrier Really Contribute?" *Neurobiology Aging, 7* (1986):510–511.

Goudsmit, J. et al. "Evidence for and against the Transmissibility of Alzheimer's Disease." *Neuro., 30* (1980):945–950.

Greenwald, B.S. et al. "Neurotransmitter Deficits in Alzheimer's Disease." *J. Amer. Geriat. Soc., 31* (1983):310–316.

Grimes, A.M. et al. "Central Auditory Function in Alzheimer's Disease." *Neuro., 35* (1985):352–358.

Gurland, B.J. "The Borderlands of Dementia: The Influence of Sociocultural Characteristics on Rats of Dementia Occurring the Senium." In *Clinical Aspects of Alzheimer's Disease and Senile Dementia (Aging,* Vol. 15), edited by Miller, N.E., and Cohen, G.D., 61–84. New York: Raven Press, 1981.

Hardy, J.A. et al. "An Integrative Hypothesis Concerning the Pathogenesis and Progression of Alzheimer's Disease." *Neurobiology of Aging, 7* (1986):489–502.

Haugen, P.K. "Behaviour of Patients with Dementia." *DMB, Gerontology, 1* (1985):62–64.

Hauser, W.A. et al. "Seizures and Myoclonus in Patients with Alzheimer's Disease." *Neuro., 36* (1986):1226–1230.

Hefti, F. "On the Pathogenesis of Alzheimer's Disease." *Neurobiology of Aging, 7* (1986):514–515.

Heinsimer, J.A., and Lefkowitz, R.J. "The Impact of Aging on Adrenergic Receptor Function." *JAGS, 3* (1985):184–188.

Henig, R. *The Myth of Senility: Misconceptions about the Brain and Aging.* Doubleday: Anchor Press, 1981.

Henry, J.P. "Relation of Psychosocial Factors to the Senile Dementias." In *The Dementias: Policy and Management,* edited by Gilhooly, M.L. et al., 38–65. New Jersey: Prentice-Hall, 1986.

Heston, L.L. *Alzheimer's Disease and Related Disorders Association Newsletter, 5* (Summer 1985).

Heston, L.L et al. "Dementia of the Alzheimer type." *Arch. Gen. Psychiatry, 38* (1981):1085-1090.

Heston, L.L., and White, J. *Dementia: A Practical Guide to Alzheimer's Disease and Related Disorders.* New York: W.H. Freeman and Co., 1983.

Heyman, A. et al. "Lecithin Therapy of Alzheimer's Disease: A Preliminary Report." In *Alzheimer's Disease: A Report of Progress in Research (Aging,* Vol. 19), edited by Corkin, S. et al., 373–378. New York: Raven Press, 1982.

Hollister, L.E., and Yesavage, J. "Ergoloid Mesylates for Senile Dementia: Unanswered Questions. *Ann. Intern. Med., 100* (1984):894–898.

Huber, S.J., and Paulson, G.W. "The Concept of Subcortical Dementia." *Am. J. Psychiatry, 142* (1985):1312–1317.

Huff, F.J. et al. "Age at Onset and Rate of Progression of Alzheimer's Disease." *JAGS, 35* (1987):27–30.

Hutton, J.T. "Evaluation and Treatment of Dementia." *Texas Med., 83* (1987):20–24.

Hyman, B.T. et al. "Alzheimer's Disease: Cell-specific Pathology Isolates the Hippocampal Formation." *Science, 225* (1984):1168–1170.

Iqbal, K., and Wisniewski, H. "Neurofibrillary Tangles." In *Alzheimer's Disease: The Standard Reference,* edited by Reisberg, B., 48–57. New York: The Free Press, 1983.

Jarvik, L.F. "Genetic Factors and Chromosomal Aberrations in Alzheimer's Disease, Senile Dementia, and Related Disorders." In *Alzheimer's Disease: Senile Dementia and Related Disorders (Aging,* Vol. 7), edited by Katzman, R. et al., 273–277. New York: Raven Press, 1978.

Jenike, M.A. *Handbook of Geriatric Psychopharmacology.* Littleton, Massachusetts: PSG Publishing Co., Inc., 1985.

Jenike, M.A. et al. "Combination Therapy with Lecithin and Ergoloid Mesylates for Alzheimer's Disease." *J. Am. Psychiatry, 47* (1986):249–251.

Jorm, A.F. "Subtypes of Alzheimer's Dementia: A Conceptual Analysis and Critical View." *Psychol. Med., 15* (1985):543–553.

Justice, B. *Who Gets Sick: Thinking and Health.* Houston, Texas: Peak Press, 1987.

Karlinsky, H. "Alzheimer's Disease in Down's Syndrome." *JAGS, 34* (1986):728–734.

Katzman, R. "Alzheimer's Disease." *N. Engl. J. Med., 314* (1986):964–973.

Kaye, W.H. et al. "Cognitive Effects of Cholinergic and Vasopressin-like Agents in Patients with Primary Degenerative Dementia." In *Alzheimer's Disease: A Report of Progress in Research (Aging,* Vol. 19), edited by Corkin, S. et al., 433–422. New York: Raven Press, 1982.

Kaye, W.H., Sitaram, N. et al. "Modest Facilitation of Memory in Dementia with Combined Lecithin and Anticholinesterase Treatment." *Biol. Psychiatry, 17* (1982):275–280.

Kemper, T. "Neuroanatomical and Neuropathological Changes in Normal Aging and in Dementia." In *Clinical Neurology of Aging,* edited by Albert, M. New York: Oxford University Press, 1984.

Kidd, M. et al. "Senile Plaque Amyloid, Paired Helical Filaments, and Cerebrovascular Amyloid in Alzheimer's Disease are all Deposits of the Same Protein." *The Lancet* (Feb. 2, 1985):278–279.

Kirshner, H.S. et al. "Language Disturbance: An Initial Symptom of Cortical Degenerations and Dementia." *Arch. Neurol., 41* (1984):491–496.

Kolata, G. "Researchers Hunt for Alzheimer's Disease Gene." *Science, 232* (1986):448–450.

Kolb, B., and Whishaw, I. *Fundamentals of Human Neuropsychology.* San Francisco: W.H. Freeman and Co., 1980.

Kopelman, M.D. "Multiple memory deficits in Alzheimer's-type dementia: Implications for pharmacotherapy." *Psychol. Med., 15* (1985):527–541.

Kral, V.A. "Benign Senescent Forgetfulness." In *Alzheimer's Disease: Senile Dementia and Related Disorders (Aging, Vol. 7)*, edited by Katzman, R. et al., 47–52. New York: Raven Press, 1978.

Kübler-Ross, E. *On Death and Dying*. New York: MacMillan, 1969, 38–137.

Laveren-Huyven, C.M.S. et al. "Double-blind clinical and Psychologic Study of Ergolois Mesylates (Hydergine) in subjects with senile mental deterioration." *JAGS, 32* (1984):584-588.

Lawton, M.P. "Sensory Deprivation and the Effect of the Environment on Management of the Patient with Senile Dementia." In *Clinical Aspects of Alzheimer's Disease and Senile Dementia (Aging, Vol. 15)*, edited by Miller, N.E., and Cohen, G.D., 227–252. New York: Raven Press, 1981.

Lazarus, L.W. et al. "Frequency and Presentation of Depressive Symptoms in Patients with Primary Degenerative Dementia." *Am. J. Psychiatry, 144* (1987):41–45.

Leffell, M.S. et al. "An Analysis of T Lymphocyte Subpopulations in Patients with Alzheimer's Disease." *JAGS, 33* (1985):4–8.

Lerer, B., and Friedman, E. "Neurochemical Lesion Models." In *Alzheimer's Disease: The Standard Reference*, edited by Reisberg, B., 369–373. New York: The Free Press, 1983.

Levy, R. "Tetrahydroaminoacridine and Alzheimer's Disease." *The Lancet* (Feb. 7, 1978):322.

Lewin, R. "Brain Grafts Benefit Parkinson's Patients." *Science, 236* (1987):149.

Lindeman, A. *Alzheimer's Disease Handbook*. San Francisco, California: Andus Older Adult Center, 1983.

Lippa, A.S., and Bartus, R.T. "Neurobiological Aspects of Geriatric Cognitive Dysfunction." In *Alzheimer's Disease: A Report of Progress in Research (Aging, Vol. 19)*, edited by Corkin, S. et al., 373–388. New York: Raven Press, 1982.

Lipowski, Z.J. "Differentiating Delirium from Dementia in the Elderly." *Clin. Geront., 1* (1982):1.

McDonald, C. "Clinical Heterogeneity in Senile Dementia." *Brit. J. Psychiat., 115* (1969):267–271.

McDuff, T., and Sumi, S.M. "Subcortical Degeneration in Alzheimer's Disease." *Neuro., 35* (1985):123–126.

McKhann, C. et al. "Clinical Diagnosis of Alzheimer's Disease: Report of the NINCDS-ADRDA Work Group Under the Auspices of Department of Health and Human Services Task Force on Alzheimer's Disease." *Neuro, 34* (1984):939–944.

McKinney, M. et al. "Cortical Cholinergic Innervation: Implications for the Pathophysiology and Treatment of Alzheimer's Disease." In *Alzheimer's Disease: A Report of Progress in Research (Aging, Vol. 19)*, edited by Corkin, S. et al., 259–266. New York: Raven Press, 1982.

Mace, N., and Rabins, P. *The 36-Hour Day*. New York: John Hopkin's University Press, 1985.

Madrazo, I. et al. "Open Microsurgical Autograft of Adrenal Medulla to the Right Caudate Nucleus in Two Patients with Intractable Parkinson's Disease." *N. Engl. J. Med., 316* (1987):831–834.

Mann, D.M.A. "Changes in Protein Synthesis," In *Alzheimer's Disease: The Standard Reference*, edited by Reisberg, B., 107–115. New York: The Free Press, 1983.

Marcer, D. "Measuring Memory Change in Alzheimer's Disease." In *Alzheimer's Disease: Early Recognition of Potentially Reversible Deficits,* edited by Glen A.I.M., and Whalley, L.J., 117–121. London and New York: Churchill Livingstone, 1979.

Masters, C.L. et al. "The Familial Occurrence of Cruetzfeldt-Jakob Disease and Alzheimer's Disease." *Brain, 104* (1981):535–558.

Masters, C.L., and Beyreuther, K. "Amyloid Filaments in Alzheimer's Disease." *Psychol. Med., 16* (1986):735–737.

Matsuyamd, H. "Incidence of Neurofibrillary Change, Senile Plaques and Granulo-vacuolar Degeneration in Aged Individuals." In *Alzheimer's Disease: The Standard Reference,* edited by Reisberg, B., 149–154. New York: The Free Press, 1983.

Matsuyama, S.S. "Genetic Factors." In *Alzheimer's Disease: The Standard Reference,* edited by Reisberg, B., 155–160. New York: The Free Press, 1983.

Mayeux, R. et al. "Heterogeneity in Dementia of the Alzheimer-type: Evidence of Subgroups." *Neuro., 35* (1985):453–461.

Merz, B. "Adrenal-to-Brain Transplants Improve the Prognosis for Parkinson's Disease." *JAMA, 257* (1987):2691–2692.

Merz, P.A. et al. "Infection-specific Particle from the Unconventional Slow Virus Diseases." *Science, 225* (1984):437–439.

Mohs, R.C., and Davies, K.L. "Cholinomimetic Drug Effects on Memory in Young and Elderly Adults." In *Alzheimer's Disease: Early Recognition of Potentially Reversible Deficits,* edited by Glen A.I.M., and Whalley, L.J., 154–158. London and New York: Churchill Livingstone, 1979.

Mohs, R.C. et al. "Defining Treatment Efficacy in Patients with Alzheimer's Disease." In *Alzheimer's Disease: A Report of Progress in Research (Aging,* Vol. 19), edited by Corkin, S. et al., 351–356. New York: Raven Press, 1982.

Mohs, R.C., and Davis, B.M. et al. "Clinical Studies of the Cholinergic Deficit in Alzheimer's Disease." *JAGS, 33* (1985):749–757.

Mölsä, P.K. et al. Extrapyramidal Signs in Alzheimer's Disease." *Neuro., 34* (1984):1114–1116.

Moore, R.Y. "Parkinson's Disease—A New Therapy?" *N. Engl. J. Med., 316* (1987):872–873.

Moore, V., and Wyke, M. "Drawing Disability in Patients with Senile Dementia." *Psychol. Med., 14* (1984):97–105.

Mortimer, J.A. "Alzheimer's Disease and Senile Dementia: Prevalence and Incidence." In *Alzheimer's Disease: The Standard Reference,* edited by Reisberg, B., 141–148. New York: The Free Press, 1983.

Mortimer, J.A. et al. "Head Injury as a Risk Factor for Alzheimer's Disease." *Neuro., 35* (1985):264–267.

Moss, D.E., and Rodriguez, L.A. "Alzheimer's Dementia: Recent Developments in Cholinergic Pharmacology." *Texas Med., 83* (1987):32–34.

Mozar, H.N. et al. "Perspectives on the Etiology of Alzheimer's disease." *JAMA, 257* (1987):1503–1507.

Nandy, K. "Brain-reactive Antibodies in Aging and Senile Dementia." In *Alzheimer's Disease: Senile Dementia and Related Disorders (Aging,* Vol. 7), edited by Katzman, R. et al., 503–512. New York: Raven Press, 1978.

Nandy K., "Immunologic Factors." In *Alzheimer's Disease: The Standard Reference*, edited by Reisberg, B., 135–138. New York: The Free Press, 1983.

Nee, L.E. et al. "A Family with Histologically Confirmed Alzheimer's Disease." *Arch. Neurol., 40* (1983):203–208.

Nee, L.E. et al. "Dementia of the Alzheimer-type: Clinical and Family Study of 22 Twin Pairs." *Neuro, 37* (1987):359–363.

National Institute of Health. *Progress Report on Senile Dementia of the Alzheimer's Type.* Publication no. 81-2343. September 1981.

Nissen, M.J. et al. "Spatial Vision in Alzheimer's Disease." *Arch. Neurol., 42* (1985):667–671.

O'Connor, J. "Drug Gets Impressive Results in Alzheimer's Patients." *Psychiatric News, 21,* no. 23 (Dec. 5, 1986):1, 7, 25.

Oliver, C., and Holland, A.J. "Down's Syndrome and Alzheimer's Disease: A Review." *Psychol. Med., 16* (1986):307–322.

Oliver, R., and Bock, F. "Alleviating the Distress of Caregivers of Alzheimer's Disease Patients: A Rational-Emotive Therapy Model." *Clinical Geronot., 3* (1985):4.

Oppeneer, J., and Vervoren, T. *Gerontological Pharmacology: A Resource for Health Practitioners.* St. Louis: C.V. Mosby Co., 1983.

Orr, N.K. et al. *The Hidden Victims of Alzheimer's Disease: Families Under Stress.* New York: New York University Press, 1985.

Peabody, C.A. et al. "Thyrotropin-releasing Hormone Stimulation Test and Alzheimer's Disease." *Biol. Psychiatry, 21* (1986):553–556.

Perl, D.P. "Pathologic Association of Aluminum in Alzheimer's Disease." In *Alzheimer's Disease: The Standard Reference,* edited by Reisberg, B., 116–122. New York: The Free Press, 1983.

Perry, E.K. "Correlations Between Psychiatric, Neuropathological and Biochemical Findings in Alzheimer's Disease." In *Alzheimer's Disease: Early Recognition of Potentially Reversible Deficits,* edited by Glen A.I.M., and Whalley, L.J., 27–32. London and New York: Churchill Livingstone, 1979.

Perry, E.K., and Perry, R.H. "Acetylcholinesterase in Alzheimer's Disease." In *Alzheimer's Disease: The Standard Reference,* edited by Reisberg, B., 93–99. New York: The Free Press, 1983.

Perry, E.K., and Perry, R.H. "A Review of Neuropathological and Neurochemical Correlates of Alzheimer's Disease." *DMB, Gerontology, 1* (1985):27–34.

Peters, B.H., and Levin, H.S. "Chronic Oral Physostigmine and Lecithin Administration in Memory Disorders of Aging." In *Alzheimer's Disease: A Report of Progress in Research (Aging,* Vol. 19), edited by Corkin, S. et al., 421–426. New York: Raven Press, 1982.

Peterson, J. "Social-psychological Aspect of Death and Dying and Mental Health." In *Handbook of Mental Health and Aging,* edited by Birren, J., and Sloane, R.B., 922–942. New Jersey: Prentice-Hall, 1980.

Pollock, N.J. et al. "Filamentous Aggregates in Pick's Disease, Progressive Supranuclear Palsy, and Alzheimer's Disease Share Antigenic Determinants with Microtubule-associated Protein, TAU," *The Lancet* (Nov. 22, 1986):1211.

Pomara, N. et al. "A Dose-response Study of Lecithin in the Treatment of Alzheimer's Disease." In *Alzheimer's Disease: A Report of Progress in*

Research (Aging, Vol. 19), edited by Corkin, S. et al., 379–384. New York: Raven Press, 1982.

Powell, L., and Courtice, K. *Alzheimer's Disease: A Guide for Families.* Reading, Massachusetts: Addison-Wiley Publishing Co., 1983.

Prien, R.F. "Psychostimulants in the Treatment of Senile Dementia." In *Alzheimer's Disease: The Standard Reference,* edited by Reisberg, B., 381–386. New York: The Free Press, 1983.

Prusiner, S.B. "Some Speculations about Prions, Amyloid, and Alzheimer's Disease." *N. Engl. J. Med., 310* (1984):661–663.

Rathbone-McCuan, E., and Hashmi, J. *Isolated Elders: Health and Social Intervention.* Rockville, Maryland: Aspen Publications, 1983.

Reifler, B.V. et al. "Dementia of the Alzheimer's type and depression." *JAGS, 34* (1986):855–859.

Reisberg, B. *A Guide to Alzheimer's Disease: For Families, Spouses and Friends.* New York: The Free Press, 1981.

Reisberg, B. (ed.) *Alzheimer's Disease: The Standard Reference.* New York: The Free Press, 1983.

Reisberg, B. et al. "Signs, Symptoms and Course of Age-associated Cognitive Decline." In *Alzheimer's Disease: A Report of Progress in Research (Aging,* Vol. 19), edited by Corkin, S. et al., 177–182. New York: Raven Press, 1982.

Reisberg, B. et al. "Effects of Naloxone in Senile Dementia." *N. Engl. J. Med., 308* (1983):721–722.

Reisberg, B., and Borenstein, J. et al. "Behavioral Symptoms in Alzheimer's Disease." *J. Clin. Psychiatry, 48* (1987):9–15.

Restak, Richard M. *The Brain.* New York: Bantam Books, 1984, 10–14, 338–342.

Rosan, R.C. "Physical Complications of Alzheimer's Disease." *Med. Aspects Human Sexuality, 21* (1987):77–88.

Rose, R.P., and Moulthrop, M.A. "Differential Responsivity of Verbal and Visual Recognition Memory to Physostigmine and ACTH." *Biol. Psychiatry, 21* (1986):538–542.

Rosen, W.G., and Mohs, R.C. "Evolution of Cognitive Decline in Dementia." In *Alzheimer's Disease: A Report of Progress in Research (Aging,* Vol. 19), edited by Corkin, S. et al., 183–188. New York: Raven Press, 1982.

Rosenberg, G.S. et al. "Pharmacologic Treatment of Alzheimer's Disease: An Overview." In *Alzheimer's Disease: The Standard Reference,* edited by Reisberg, B., 329–339. New York: The Free Press, 1983.

Rossor, M.N. et al. "Neuropeptides and Neurotransmitters in Cerebral Cortex in Alzheimer's Disease." In *Alzheimer's Disease: A Report of Progress in Research (Aging,* Vol. 19), edited by Corkin, S. et al., 15–24. New York: Raven Press, 1982.

Rossor, M.N., and Garrett, N.J. et al. "A Post-mortem Study of the Cholinergic and GABA Systems in Senile Dementia." *Brain, 105* (1982):313–330.

Rossor, M.N., and Iversen, L.L. et al. "Neurochemical Characteristics of Early and Late Onset Types of Alzheimer's Disease." *Brit. Med. J., 228* (1984):961–964.

Roth, M. "Diagnosis of Senile and Related Forms of Dementia." In *Alzheimer's Disease: Senile Dementia and Related Disorders (Aging,* Vol. 7), edited by Katzman, R. et al., 71–86. New York: Raven Press, 1978.

Salazar, A.M. et al. "Relation to Creutzfeldt-Jakob Disease and Other Unconventional Virus Diseases." In *Alzheimer's Disease: The Standard Reference,* edited by Reisberg, B., 311–318. New York: The Free Press, 1983.

Saper, C.B. et al. "Neuronal Pathology in the Nucleus Basalis and Associated Cell Groups in Senile Dementia of the Alzheimer Type." *Neuro., 35* (1985):1089–1095.

Schmeck, Harold. "Blood Abnormality May Predict Alzheimer's." *The New York Times* (October 29, 1987).

Schneck, M.K. "Nootropics." In *Alzheimer's Disease: The Standard Reference,* edited by Reisberg, B., 362–368. New York: The Free Press, 1983.

Selkoe, D.J. et al. "Conservation of Brain Amyloid Proteins in Aged Mammals and Humans with Alzheimer's Disease." *Science, 235* (1987):873–877.

Seltzer, B., and Sherrwin, I. "A Comparison of Clinical Features in Early- and Late-Onset Primary Degenerative Dementia." *Arch. Neurol., 40* (1983):143–146.

Shore, P., and Wyatt, R.J. "Aluminum and Alzheimer's Disease." *J. Nervous Ment. Disease, 171* (1983):353–558.

Sims, N.R., and Bowen, D.M. et al. "Biochemical Changes in Cortical Brain Biopsies from Demented Patients." In *Alzheimer's Disease: A Report of Progress in Research (Aging,* Vol. 19), edited by Corkin, S. et al., 1–8. New York: Raven Press, 1982.

Sims, N.R., and Bowen, D.M. "Changes in Choline Acetyltransferase and in Acetylcholine Synthesis." In *Alzheimer's Disease: The Standard Reference,* edited by Reisberg, B., 88–92. New York: The Free Press, 1983.

Sitaram, N., and Weingartner, H. "Cholinergic Mechanisms in Human Memory." In *Alzheimer's Disease: Early Recognition of Potentially Reversible Deficits,* edited by Glen A.I.M., and Whalley, L.J., 159–162. London and New York: Churchill Livingstone, 1979.

Sitaram, N. et al. "Combination Treatment of Alzheimer's Dementia." In *Alzheimer's Disease: The Standard Reference,* edited by Reisberg, B., 355–361. New York: The Free Press, 1983.

Smith, C.M. et al. "Effects of Cholinergic Drugs on Memory in Alzheimer's Disease." In *Alzheimer's Disease: Early Recognition of Potentially Reversible Deficits,* edited by Glen A.I.M., and Whalley, L.J., 148–153. London and New York: Churchill Livingstone, 1978.

Smith, C.M., and Semple, S.A. "Effects of Physostigmine on Responses in Memory Tests in Patients with Alzheimer's Disease." In *Alzheimer's Disease: A Report of Progress in Research (Aging,* Vol. 19), edited by Corkin, S. et al., 405–412. New York: Raven Press, 1982.

Soininen, H. et al. "Treatment of Alzheimer's Disease with Synthetic ACTH 4-9 Analog." *Neuro., 35* (1985):1348–1351.

Spence, M.A. et al. "Genetic Linkage Studies in Alzheimer's Disease." *Neuro., 36* (1986):581–584.

St. George-Hyslop, P.H. et al. "The Genetic Defect Causing Familial Alzheimer's Disease Maps on Chromosome 21." *Science, 235* (1987):885–889.

Steffes, R., and Thralow, J. "Visual Field Limitation in the Patient with the Dementia of the Alzheimer's Type." *JAGS, 35* (1987):198–204.

Stipp, D. "New Findings about Alzheimer's May Offer Insights into its Cause." *The Wall Street Journal* (Feb. 20, 1987):21.

Struble, R.G. et al. "Cholinergic Innervation in Neuritic Plaques." *Science, 216* (1982):413–415.

Sullivan, E. et al. "Physostigmine and Lecithin in Alzheimer's Disease." In *Alzheimer's Disease: A Report of Progress in Research (Aging, Vol. 19)*, edited by Corkin, S. et al., 361–368. New York: Raven Press, 1982.

Summers, W.K. et al. Oral Tetrahydroaminoacridine in Long-term Treatment of Senile Dementia." *N. Engl. J. Med., 315* (1986):1242–1245.

Taber's Cyclopedic Medical Dictionary ed. by Thomas C., 15th edition. Philadelphia: F.A. Davis Company, 1985.

Tagliavini, F., and Pilleri, G. "Neuronal Counts in Basal Nucleus of Meynert in Alzheimer's Disease." *The Lancet* (Feb. 26, 1983):469–470.

Tamminga, N.L. et al. "Alzheimer's Disease: Low Cerebral Somatostatin Levels Correlate with Impaired Cognitive Function and Cortical Metabolism." *Neurology, 37* (1987):161–165.

Tanzi, R.E., and Gusella, J.F. et al. "Amyloid Beta-Protein Gene: cDNA, Distribution, and Genetic Linkage Near the Alzheimer Locus." *Science, 235* (1987):880–884.

Tariot, P.N., and Sunderland, T. et al. "Naloxone and Alzheimer's Disease: Cognitive and Behavioral Effects of a Range of Doses." *Arch. Gen. Psychiatry, 43* (1986):727–732.

Terry, R. "Some Unanswered Questions about the Mechanisms and Etiology of Alzheimer's Disease." *DMB, Gerontology, 1* (1985):22–24.

Terry, R. "Aging, Senile Dementia, and Alzheimer's Disease." In *Alzheimer's Disease: Senile Dementia and Related Disorders (Aging, Vol. 7)*, edited by Katzman, R. et al., 11–14. New York: Raven Press, 1978.

Teusink, J.P., and Mahler, S. "Helping Families Cope with Alzheimer's Disease." *Hospital and Community Psychiatry, 35* (1984):152–156.

Thal, L., and Fuld, P. "Memory Enhancement with Oral Physostigmine in Alzheimer's Disease." *N. Engl. J. Med., 308* (1983):720.

Thienhaus, O.J. et al. "Biologic Markers in Alzheimer's Disease." *JAGS, 33,* no. 10 (1985):715–726.

Tomlinson, B.E. "Editorial: Plaques, Tangles and Alzheimer's Disease." *Psychol. Med., 12* (1982):449–459.

Tower, D.B. "Alzheimer's Disease, Senile Dementia and Related Disorders: Neurobiological Status." In *Alzheimer's Disease: Senile Dementia and Related Disorders (Aging, Vol. 7)*, edited by Katzman, R. et al., 1–4. New York: Raven Press, 1978.

U.S. Department of Health and Human Services. *Alzheimer's Disease: A Scientific Guide for Health Practitioners.* Publication no. 81-2251, 1980.

Volicer, L. et al. "Serotoninergic System in Dementia of the Alzheimer Type." *Arch. Neurol., 42* (Dec. 85):1158–1161.

Wade, John P.H. et al. "The Clinical Diagnosis of Alzheimer's Disease." *Arch. Neurol., 44* (Jan. 1987):24–29.

Walford, R.L., and Fortoul, T. "Histocompatibility Locus Antigens and Alzheimer's Disease." In *Alzheimer's Disease: The Standard Reference,* edited by Reisberg, B., 166–170. New York: The Free Press, 1983.

Weintraub, S. et al. "Lecithin in the Treatment of Alzheimer's Disease." *Arch. Neurol., 40* (Aug. 1983):525–528.

Whalley, L.J., and Buckton, K.E. "Genetic factors in Alzheimer's Disease." In *Alzheimer's Disease: Early Recognition of Potentially Reversible Deficits,* edited by Glen A.I.M., and Whalley, L.J., 36–41. London and New York: Churchill Livingstone, 1979.

White, J.A. et al. "Fertility and Parental Age in Alzheimer's Disease." *J. Geron., 41,* no. 1 (1986):40–43.

Whitehouse, P.J. et al. "Alzheimer's disease and Senile Dementia: Loss of Neurons in the Basal Forebrain." *Science, 215* (March 5, 1982):1237–1239.

Whitford, G.M. "Alzheimer's Disease and Serotonin: A Review." *Neuropsychobiology, 15* (1986):133–142.

Winblad, B. et al. "Biogenic Amines in Brains of Patients with Alzheimer's Disease." In *Alzheimer's Disease: A Report of Progress in Research (Aging,* Vol. 19), edited by Corkin, S. et al., 25–34. New York: Raven Press, 1982.

Winogrond, I.R., and Fisk, A.A. "Alzheimer's Disease: Assessment of Functional Status." *J. of Amer. Geri. Soc., 31,* no. 12 (Dec. 1983):780–785.

Wisniewski, H.M. "Possible Viral Etiology of Neurofibrillary Changes and Neuritic Plaques." In *Alzheimer's Disease: Senile Dementia and Related Disorders (Aging,* Vol. 7), edited by Katzman, R. et al., 555–558. New York: Raven Press, 1978.

Wisniewski, H.M. "Neurofibrillary and Synaptic Pathology in Senile Dementia of the Alzheimer's Type." In *Alzheimer's Disease: Early Recognition of Potentially Reversible Deficits,* edited by Glen A.I.M., and Whalley, L.J., 7–16. London and New York: Churchill Livingstone, 1979.

Wisniewski, H.M. "Neuritic (Senile) and Amyloid Plaques." In *Alzheimer's Disease: The Standard Reference,* edited by Reisberg, B., 57–61. New York: The Free Press, 1983.

Wisniewski, K.E. et al. "Age-associated Changes and Dementia in Down's Syndrome." In *Alzheimer's Disease: The Standard Reference,* edited by Reisberg, B., 319–326. New York: The Free Press, 1983.

Wurtman, R.J. "Forecast." In *Alzheimer's Disease: A Report of Progress in Research (Aging,* Vol. 19), edited by Corkin, S. et al., 495–500. New York: Raven Press, 1982.

Yates, C.M. "Aluminum and Alzheimer's Disease." In *Alzheimer's Disease: Early Recognition of Potentially Reversible Deficits,* edited by Glen A.I.M., and Whalley, L.J., 53–56. London and New York: Churchill Livingstone, 1979.

Yesavage, J.A. "Use of Vasoactive Medications in the Treatment of Senile Dementia." In *Alzheimer's Disease: The Standard Reference,* edited by Reisberg, B., 374–380. New York: The Free Press, 1983.

Zarit, S. et al. *The Hidden Victims of Alzheimer's Disease: Families Under Stress.* New York: University Press, 1985.

Zarit, S., and Zarit, J. *Working with Families of Dementia Victims: A Treatment Manual.* Los Angeles: Andrew Older Adult Center, 1983.

Zarit, S., and Zarit, J. "Cognitive Impairment." In *Clinical Geropsychology: New Directions in Assessment and Treatment,* edited by Lewinsohn, P. and Teri, L. New York: Pergamon Press, 1983., 38–80.

INDEX